Coping with

I0056736

LYME DISEASE

Karen Donnelly

The Rosen Publishing Group, Inc.
New York

To my husband, David, and to my beautiful and brilliant daughters, Cathy and especially Colleen, who suffered through the arthritic symptoms of Lyme disease when she was seven years old.

Published in 2001 by The Rosen Publishing Group, Inc.
29 East 21st Street, New York, NY 10010

Copyright © 2001 by Karen Donnelly

First Edition

Cover photo © Archive Photography

Library of Congress Cataloging-in-Publication Data

Donnelly, Karen.
    Coping with Lyme disease / by Karen Donnelly — 1st ed.
        p.   cm.
    Includes bibliographical references and index.
    ISBN: 978-1-4358-8648-3
    1. Lyme disease—Juvenile literature.   [1. Lyme disease. 2. Diseases.] I. Title.
    RC155.5 .D659   2000
    616.9'2—dc21   00-009909
                                                              CIP
                                                              AC

Manufactured in the United States of America

About the Author

Karen Donnelly, a writer from Connecticut, has a master's degree in English literature from Southern Connecticut State University. She has written numerous books and newspaper and magazine articles for children and adults on such topics as nature, architecture, careers, and health.

Contents

Introduction

At the end of the twentieth century, Lyme disease had two faces. On the one hand, Lyme disease was easily recognized and treated. A telltale rash announced its presence. A course of oral antibiotics successfully treated the infection.

But a second face was masked. No rash appeared and the bacteria that caused the infection spread throughout the body. An accompanying slight fever and general achiness may have been attributed to the flu. As time went on, joint pain and stiffness would result and were usually attributed to arthritis. The central nervous system (CNS) and major organs were affected, but the source was not known. Symptoms worsened, perhaps resulting in tremors, loss of memory, extreme fatigue, and recurring headaches. Treatments failed. Patients were accused of making up their symptoms. Some were referred to psychiatrists.

Over the years, doctors have learned more and more about Lyme disease. They are more likely to recognize a widening variety of extreme symptoms as being possibly caused by Lyme disease and to suggest that their patients get tested for the illness. But in the past, many people suffered from undiagnosed Lyme disease. They often received unnecessary treatments that did nothing to control the true cause of their symptoms. Instead, the bacteria that caused their infection spread throughout their bodies, causing serious harm. Sometimes, people died—not necessarily from the infection itself, but from the damage the disease did to their bodies. In a few cases, Lyme disease may have caused the deaths of babies born to pregnant women infected with Lyme disease.

Lyme disease, even today, is mysterious and methods of treatment are controversial. But doctors do know more now than ever before, and prospects for cures and treatments are being rigorously tested. One thing is certain: The best defense against this strange and debilitating illness is knowledge about early signs of the disease and prevention.

The Mysterious Disease Identified

In the United States, many people believe that Lyme disease is a new phenomenon, but that is not completely true. The infection that the Lyme bacteria causes has been around for a very long time. In 1883, a German doctor named Alfred Buchwald first described a skin disorder resembling what we now call erythema migrans (EM), the "bull's eye" rash common with Lyme disease. But Dr. Buchwald and other scientists of his time did not connect the rash to other more severe symptoms. Even when doctors realized that patients with EM rashes also had symptoms like joint pain or severe headaches, they still did not connect it to Lyme disease.

A Mysterious Disease

Peggy Wilson was sick and she didn't know why. Sometimes she thought she was going crazy.

The first time Peggy went to see Dr. Monroe, she complained of severe headaches. She also had sharp pains in her right elbow and her back.

"Dr. Monroe," Peggy said, "these headaches seem to appear from nowhere. My head hurts so much I have to stop what I'm doing. Sometimes I feel like

screaming. At home, I can lie down until the pain passes. But if I get one while I'm at work, I have to stay in the ladies' room. I can't talk to anyone."

"Do the headaches happen more often at work or at home?" asked Dr. Monroe.

"At work, I guess," said Peggy.

"Are you under any added pressure at work? Has something changed there?" Dr. Monroe asked.

"Well, yes," said Peggy. "Since the layoffs, we have to do the same amount of work with three people instead of four. When we're nearing a deadline, it can get pretty hectic. If we complain, my boss just keeps repeating, 'We'll make the deadline. There are no other options.'"

"There's the cause of your headaches, Peggy," said Dr. Monroe. "I'll prescribe some pills for you that will help with the pain. I think you just have to ride them out until your work situation improves."

"What about my elbow?" asked Peggy. "Sometimes I can't even lift a gallon of milk. And some mornings my back hurts so much I can hardly get out of bed. That can't be caused by stress."

"Tension in your muscles could be causing your joint and back pain," said Dr. Monroe. "Your elbow pain could be caused by injury. Do you remember lifting anything that could have pulled your arm back too far? Sometimes the pain does not begin right away so it's hard to associate with the actual injury."

"Sometimes I have to lift Carrie, my niece, out of her car seat," said Peggy. "It's a bit awkward because I'm leaning into the backseat of the car."

"That's likely the cause," said Dr. Monroe. "You have probably stressed your elbow and your back repeatedly and now it has become painful. The next time you take Carrie out of her car seat, think about how you carry her and try not to bend in awkward positions."

"I'll try," said Peggy.

Before the 1970s, people in the Unites States suffered from Lyme disease, but no one knew it. Doctors had not identified the disease or the bacteria that caused it. So sometimes people who suffered from Lyme disease were diagnosed with other illnesses, like the flu or multiple sclerosis. Sometimes they were told that their symptoms were psychosomatic, or in their heads. Their doctors thought that the patients were not really sick, but were imagining or exaggerating their symptoms.

Doctors told Polly Murray her symptoms were not real, but she knew that the doctors were wrong. Polly lived in Lyme, Connecticut. She had been sick on and off for more than ten years. Her head and neck ached. A rash appeared on her hands, disappeared, then appeared again. She had terrible pain in her joints and sometimes had to keep her arm in a sling. Over the years, she was tested for many diseases, but doctors could never find the cause of her symptoms.

In the summer of 1975, Polly and her entire family were very sick. Her husband had difficulty speaking because he had laryngitis. His knees were swollen and so painful that he had to walk with crutches. Her sons seemed to have juvenile rheumatoid arthritis, a disease that causes children to have stiff, painful joints. One son also had vision problems. Her daughter's tongue swelled so much that she almost missed her high school graduation. They also had bizarre rashes. At times, their symptoms would seem to be cured, but then the pain came back. Even their dog was sick.

The Mystery Is Uncovered

Polly knew something was terribly wrong, but the doctors she took her family to could not help them. She looked everywhere for causes. She thought that perhaps her water had been polluted. But when she had the water tested, it was fine.

Polly began talking to her neighbors. She discovered that many of them had also been sick with the same mysterious symptoms. Finally, in October 1975, she contacted the Connecticut Health Department. She was referred to Dr. Allen C. Steere, then a doctor at Yale University. Dr. Steere was interested in studying arthritis. Arthritis was not considered to be a contagious disease, but Dr. Steere thought it might be possible to "catch" it. In order to test his theory, he needed to find a group of people in a small geographical area who had arthritis. He would try to learn how all these people got the disease.

Dr. Steere and his colleagues began seeing and talking to people in Lyme, Connecticut, who had stiff and swollen joints. By May 1976, they had found thirty-nine children and twelve adults who lived in or near Lyme and seemed to have arthritis. Dr. Steere believed that he had discovered a new kind of arthritis and named it "Lyme arthritis" after the town. Later, as doctors realized that these people were suffering from many symptoms other than arthritis, the name was changed to Lyme disease.

Scientists and doctors still needed more information. They did not know what caused Lyme disease or how to treat it. Soon, Dr. Steere began to suspect tick bites. But it was not until 1979 that the deer tick, or blacklegged tick, was identified as the carrier of the Lyme disease bacteria by Dr. Andrew Spielman. Questions still remained, however. What kind of germ causes the infection? How does the infection get from a tick to a human?

Dr. Willy Burgdorfer and Dr. Jorge Benach had been studying a different disease called Rocky Mountain spotted fever on Long Island. They believed that this disease might also be caused by ticks. When they looked at bacteria carried by deer ticks, they discovered that the bacteria did not cause Rocky Mountain spotted fever. But they did find a strange kind of bacteria, called a spirochete, in deer ticks.

They checked blood samples taken from Lyme disease patients and found that the samples also contained the spirochete type of bacteria. In 1984, the bacteria was named *Borrelia burgdorferi*, after Dr. Burgdorfer. The bacteria can be seen only under a microscope. If you laid 100,000 *Borrelia burgdorferi* side by side, they would fill about an inch of space. Since the bacteria were first discovered, about 100 different strains, or types, have been found in the United States.

Studies continued and now doctors know a lot more about Lyme disease and how to treat it. They know that antibiotics will probably cure someone who gets treatment right away, within six weeks of being bitten by a tick. Problems arise, however, when the infection goes untreated. This can happen frequently because tick bites do not hurt. You probably would not feel a tick bite you.

Many people who are later diagnosed with Lyme disease cannot remember being bitten. The telltale sign, an EM rash, appears only 60 to 70 percent of the time. Early diagnosis for people who do not have this rash is very difficult.

Left untreated, Lyme disease can have very serious consequences. Some people, especially those who suffered with Lyme disease before doctors knew what it was or how to treat it, still have very severe health problems today.

Peggy Wilson took Dr. Monroe's advice, but her symptoms did not improve. In fact, they worsened. She was tired all the time. The pain in her elbow had gone away for a while, but now it was back. Her knees were swollen and painful, too. She had a rash on her arm. When her hands began to tremble for no apparent reason, she went back to Dr. Monroe.

"Has your job situation improved, Peggy?" asked Dr. Monroe.

"There's still a lot of stress, but I don't think that's the real problem," said Peggy. "In fact, if we don't find out what the real problem is, I may not have a job to worry about. I've had to take unpaid days off because I used up all my sick days. My boss is getting tired of this and so am I."

"Worrying about getting fired may just be adding to the pressure you're under," said Dr. Monroe.

"Look," said Peggy. "I don't believe that my symptoms are caused just by stress. I think there's something really wrong with me. And while you're prescribing pain medication, I'm just getting worse. I want some real answers."

Symptoms: From
Rashes to Arthritis

Ticks, mice, and deer carry bacteria called *Borrelia burgdorferi*. This thin, spiral kind of bacteria is called a spirochete. When a tick that is carrying the *Borrelia burgdorferi* bacteria bites you, it infects your bloodstream with the bacteria. If it is left untreated, the bacteria can travel all over your body. It usually attacks your joints and nervous system.

Stage I Lyme Disease

Each June, Nathan Melton spent a week with his cousins, aunt, and uncle on Long Beach Island in New Jersey. Their house was right on the beach. Nathan could step out the door and run straight into the waves. His uncle also docked a motorboat at the marina. Nathan loved to take the boat for a ride with his cousins in the bay. Sometimes his uncle drove the boat, and Nathan, his aunt, and his cousins would take turns waterskiing.

Nathan also liked to explore the marsh. He was an avid photographer. He hid in the tall grass to get close-up shots of birds and other wildlife. After the hectic school year, a quiet week along the water was a welcome change.

Soon, though, the week was over. A few days after he got home, while he was taking a shower, Nathan noticed a strange, red rash under his arm. He had no idea what it was. It didn't look anything like the poison ivy he had last summer. He decided to show the rash to his dad.

"Dad, I have this really weird rash on my arm. It looks like it has rings, almost like a target," Nathan said. "Do you know what it is?"

Nathan's dad looked at the rash. "No, but it's really strange looking," he said. "Does it itch or hurt?"

"No," Nathan said.

"Do you feel all right otherwise?" his dad asked.

"Well, I'm tired and my head hurts a little," Nathan said. "I thought I was just worn down from all the waterskiing."

"Well, you may be right, but I think a trip to the doctor would be a good idea just to be sure," Nathan's dad said.

The first noticeable symptom of Lyme disease is often an expanding skin rash called erythema migrans, or EM, which means "wandering redness." An EM rash can be recognized in the following ways:

- ➾ It is usually lighter in the center, where the tick actually bit you. The bite spot is surrounded by darker, red rings. The rash begins small and then expands outward from the bite. These rings have given the rash its nickname, the "bull's eye" rash. Sometimes, though, the entire rash is solid red.

➥ The rash shows up usually within one to two weeks after you have been bitten (the range is from three to thirty days). That means that the Lyme disease bacteria has already been sent into your bloodstream. In fact, researchers have found that the Lyme bacteria may already have reached your spinal fluid at this time.

➥ The rash can be from two to twenty-four inches in diameter. Five to six inches is the average size. It usually lasts for about three to five weeks.

➥ An EM rash is not painful or itchy, although it may feel warm to the touch.

On light-skinned people, an EM rash is easy to see. But on people with dark or suntanned skin, the rash may look like a bruise. The EM rash is the clearest and most recognizable sign that you have been bitten by a tick and infected with the Lyme disease bacteria. Along with the rash, you may have a slight fever, a mild headache, and general achiness. These early, or Stage I, symptoms are very much like those of the flu.

Unfortunately, the rash does not appear in 30 to 40 percent of Lyme disease cases. Often, people who do not see a rash will assume their aches and fever are caused by the flu. Because the symptoms are mild, they may not even go to the doctor. Other times, because the rash does not hurt or itch, people who see the rash will not be worried and will not go to the doctor. By the time they do become concerned and make an appointment to see a doctor, the rash may have disappeared. Without this symptom, a correct diagnosis will be much more difficult. In these cases, treatment may not begin until the Lyme disease bacteria has spread and begins to cause more severe and sometimes permanently damaging problems.

Stage II, or Disseminated, Lyme Disease

One Saturday afternoon, Suzanne and Ed Lipton noticed that their daughter Claire was having trouble walking.

"Claire, why are you limping?" Ed asked. "Does your leg hurt?"

"It's my knee," said Claire. "It's swollen and really sore. I guess I must have hurt it when I went running."

"Why don't you put some ice on it and see if that helps? It should keep down the swelling," said Suzanne.

Claire iced her knee, but it didn't seem to do much good. In fact, her knee just kept getting more and more painful. By the next morning, it was so swollen and sore that she could not get up.

Panicked, Claire cried out for her mom and dad, who were making breakfast in the kitchen. What was she going to do? The big cross-country race was in just two weeks.

Claire's parents came running. They, too, were upset when they saw their daughter crying and unable to get out of bed. "I'll help her get dressed while you call Dr. Whiting," said Suzanne. "We need to get Claire to his office right away."

In children, the most common symptom of Stage II, or disseminated, Lyme disease, or Lyme disease that has spread, is painful, swollen joints, a kind of arthritis. In children, knees are affected by this Lyme arthritis more than 90 percent of the time, according to a study in the *Journal of Pediatrics*.

Lyme arthritis can come on very quickly. In twenty-four hours, you may go from feeling fine to being unable to walk. If you have not seen the EM rash, you may find yourself trying to think of a recent time that you hurt your knee. "Did I bruise my knee when I fell while skating?" "Did I twist my knee playing basketball?" Because most people are unaware of this symptom of Lyme disease, they often go searching for other causes for their pain or sickness. For this reason, people suffering from Lyme disease are often misdiagnosed.

Dr. Whiting examined Claire's knee. He gently pressed against the swelling. "Does this hurt?" he asked.

"Ow! Yes," said Claire.

"Does it hurt if you try to bend it?" he asked.

Claire tried to bend her knee. "Yes, it hurts," she said.

"I need to ask you some questions that may seem unrelated to your knee pain," said Dr. Whiting. "I know you're on the cross-country team. Do you ever go trail running?"

"Yes," Claire answered. "I run on the mountain at least three times a week and sometimes go hiking on the weekends if I don't have a race," she said.

"Are the trails clear of brush, or do you brush up against bushes and tall grass?"

"I'm always running through grass and getting scratched by branches," she said. "Sometimes I even like to run off the trail if I can."

"And what do you usually wear when you go running?" asked Dr. Whiting.

"Usually shorts and a tank top," said Claire.

"Well, the good news is that I don't think you have an injury," said Dr. Whiting. "But I think that you might have Lyme disease.

"You get infected with Lyme disease from a tick bite," he continued. "Ticks live in grass, so you could have picked one up when you brushed up against the foliage along the trail. Ticks are very small, so you may never have noticed it."

"Don't you get a rash if you have Lyme disease?" asked Claire.

"Not always," said Dr. Whiting. "And when you don't get the rash, you can have the Lyme bacteria in your body for months without being aware of it. Then suddenly, your joints swell up. Most often, knees are affected, like yours."

"I'd like you to take Claire to the hospital," Dr. Whiting said to Suzanne. "We need to give her a blood test to be sure my diagnosis is correct. Then she can begin intravenous antibiotic treatment."

Lyme disease can also affect your nervous system, which may cause a stiff neck or severe headaches. The muscles in your face may become paralyzed, making one side of your face look droopy, a condition called Bell's palsy. These symptoms usually occur several weeks or months after having become infected with the bacteria and leaving it untreated.

Stephanie spent her summer vacations on Cape Cod in Massachusetts. She worked as a lifeguard on the beach in Wellfleet. One day, near the end of July, the right side of her face felt a bit numb. As she watched swimmers bouncing in the waves, she found herself unconsciously touching her face.

"Steph, is something wrong?" asked her friend Nicole. "You keep rubbing your face."

"I don't know. It just feels funny," said Stephanie. "It's probably nothing."

The rest of the day passed normally. But the next morning, Stephanie discovered that the numbness on her face was not just "nothing." Something was really wrong!

Stephanie went into the bathroom to brush her teeth. When she looked in the mirror, she let out a shriek.

"Mom!" Stephanie yelled. "Come here. Look at my face!"

Stephanie's mom rushed to the bathroom. "What's wrong? Oh my!" she exclaimed as she entered the bathroom.

The right side of Stephanie's face looked as if it was drooping. Stephanie could not control her facial muscles. She could not pull her face back to normal. She started to panic.

"What's wrong with me?" cried Stephanie.

"I don't know, Steph," said her mom. "I'll call Dr. Hemingway and we'll go see him right away."

"Okay," answered Stephanie. "And please call Nicole. I'm supposed to guard today. Maybe she can get Mitch to cover for me."

Dr. Hemingway took one look at Stephanie and said, "That looks like Bell's palsy, a very common symptom of Lyme disease. Do you remember finding a tick on your body?"

"No, gross!" answered Stephanie.

"Do you remember seeing a red rash anywhere. The rash may have looked like a bull's eye and gotten bigger over a few days."

"No, I never had a rash," said Stephanie.

"That's unusual. As you probably know, you get Lyme disease from a tick bite," said Dr. Hemingway. "Oftentimes patients who have been infected with Lyme disease develop a rash like the one I described. But not everyone gets the rash. So you could still have Lyme disease.

"Let's talk about how you feel now. Are you having any trouble hearing?" asked Dr. Hemingway.

"No," said Stephanie.

"How about taste? When you ate breakfast did the food taste like it usually does?"

"I wasn't hungry," said Stephanie. "I didn't eat any breakfast. I was too upset. But yesterday food tasted normal."

"I'm going to run some tests," said Dr. Hemingway. "But I believe that your facial palsy is caused by a Lyme disease infection. I'm going to give you a prescription for antibiotics, pills that you should take twice a day for two weeks. Your face should return to its normal shape before long."

16

"How long will it take?" asked Stephanie.
"Total recovery could take a month or two," said Dr.
Hemingway. "But you will begin to get better shortly."
"I hope it's better by Labor Day," said Stephanie.
"I'll die if I have to start college with a droopy face."

While the symptoms we have discussed so far are the most recognizable, people with Lyme disease, especially adults, can have many other symptoms. Lyme disease has been called "the great imitator" because it can appear to be so many other diseases, making it difficult for doctors to diagnose. Stage II Lyme disease can also include the following symptoms:

- ➾ Reappearance of the same flulike symptoms experienced in Stage I of the disease, including severe headache, nausea, extreme fatigue, and vomiting

- ➾ Loss of appetite and diarrhea

- ➾ Confusion and/or temporary loss of memory

- ➾ Extreme irritability

- ➾ Extreme sensitivity to light, so that all but the dimmest light is painful

- ➾ Partial loss of vision

- ➾ Loss of smell, or extreme sensitivity to smell

- Ringing in the ear or partial hearing loss

- Tingling or numbness in fingers and toes

- Dizziness and inability to concentrate

- Loss of coordination

- Inflammation of the heart

- Swollen lymph glands

- Difficulty breathing

- Mood swings

- Difficulty sleeping

- Unexplained weight gain or loss

- Unusually great susceptibility to infection

- Tremors or unexplained shaking

- Erratic heart rhythm

Lyme disease symptoms may also migrate: They may move from one part of your body to another. They may seem to lessen, creating the impression that a treatment is working, and then return or become more severe.

Lyme disease, "the great imitator," causes symptoms very similar to several other diseases

Multiple sclerosis   This chronic disease affects the central nervous system and causes physical weakness, fatigue, memory loss, and other neurological symptoms.

Amyotrophic lateral sclerosis   This disease is also known as Lou Gehrig's disease because it was responsible for the famous baseball player's death. In its early stages, the neurological weakness it causes in arms and legs can be confused with Lyme disease.

Systemic lupus   Like Lyme disease, the symptoms of lupus may seem to lessen and worsen. Lupus affects the nervous system and may also cause fatigue and arthritis.

Infectious mononucleosis   "Mono" is caused by a virus called Epstein-Barr. It is characterized by chronic fatigue and also causes sore throat, swollen glands, and fever.

Chronic fatigue syndrome (CFS)   As the name suggests, people with CFS feel unusually tired and fatigue easily. Their disease makes going to school or work very difficult. Like mononucleosis, CFS is caused by a virus.

At the hospital, Claire and her parents waited in an examining room.

"Hello, Claire. I'm Dr. Connolly," the doctor said as she entered the room. "I've spoken to Dr. Whiting, and he told me that he suspects you may have Lyme disease. We need to take some blood from your arm. Then we'll run some tests."

"I hate needles," said Claire.

"Unfortunately, most people do," said Dr. Connolly. "Claire, please look at your mom. Keep looking at her until you feel a sharp pinch in your arm. Ready? Take a deep breath."

"Ow," said Claire.

"Keep looking at your mom," said Dr. Connolly.

Dr. Connolly used a needle with a replaceable vial that allowed her to take enough blood to run the tests without taking the needle out of Claire's arm.

"All done," said Dr. Connolly. "Have a rest for a minute. I'll send these samples to the lab so they can run the Lyme test as soon as possible. I also need to use a needle to take some of the fluid that's causing the swelling around your knee.

"Testing the fluid will ensure us that the swelling is not caused by an infection," said Dr. Connolly.

"Great," said Claire sarcastically. "More needles."

Stage III Chronic Lyme Disease

In junior high, Allison had been an honor student and captain of the swim team. But in high school, she was unable to try out for the team. Now, nearing the end of her sophomore year, Allison was forced to take remedial classes. Her Lyme disease seemed to have taken over her life.

Allison's symptoms had changed over time. Her joints, especially her knees, hurt. Sometimes she felt dizzy. She had trouble concentrating on anything. Bright lights hurt her eyes. Sometimes she had severe headaches or nausea.

Allison had gone to lots of doctors and had lots of tests. She had taken medicine orally and intravenously. Sometimes her symptoms improved and Allison thought she was finally getting better. Then the symptoms returned. Sometimes they were even worse than they had been before. The pain moved from one part of her body to another. Sometimes her neck hurt; sometimes her ankles hurt. Sometimes her hands hurt so much she could not hold a pencil or use a computer.

Stage III, or chronic, Lyme disease has become a controversial issue among doctors and patients. Symptoms that seem to have disappeared recur and worsen. Chronic arthritis, especially of the knees, sets in. Pain and swelling make walking difficult and may last for a few days or weeks, then seem to heal. But the symptoms return, over and over, sometimes for years. In this chronic stage, any of the Stage II symptoms may return and worsen, again and again.

Doctors, however, are not all in agreement about this stage of the disease. Dr. Allen C. Steere, now of Tufts University, was a pioneer in the original discovery of Lyme disease in 1975. He now believes that many people who complain of chronic Lyme disease do not actually have

Lyme disease anymore. In the *Journal of the American Medical Association* in 1993, Dr. Steere said that the illness is overdiagnosed and overtreated. He believes that the continuing symptoms are what he calls "post-Lyme syndrome." Post-Lyme syndrome involves symptoms that were caused by the damage that Lyme disease did to a person's body, which usually includes damage to the nervous and immune systems. Unlike actual Lyme disease, these symptoms are no longer being caused by the Lyme bacteria but have become separate health issues in their own right. Making this distinction is very important when deciding on the best form of treatment. Dr. Steere believes that long-term use of antibiotics—the common treatment for Lyme disease, both short-term and chronic—is not the answer for treating the symptoms associated with chronic Lyme disease. Using his studies for support, some insurance companies have refused to pay for long-term antibiotic treatment when it is prescribed for Lyme disease.

Lyme Carditis

When Lyme disease affects your heart, it is called Lyme carditis. Studies show that Lyme carditis can affect from 4 to 10 percent of people suffering from Stage III Lyme disease. Males are more likely to be affected than females.

Matt was the star of the Bethel High School varsity basketball team. He was six feet tall and very strong. He also ran track in the spring. Distance was his specialty.
Tonight, Matt was looking forward to the opening game of the basketball season. He loved to begin the

season at home. All his friends would be there, including his girlfriend, Tanya. His parents always came, too. Matt liked for his parents to watch him play, although he always pretended that he didn't care.

During the first half, Matt and his teammates were a bit nervous. They missed some baskets that they should have made. Turnovers were a problem. But their opponent, Woodrow Wilson High, was not a strong team. At the half, Bethel was ahead by five points.

During halftime, Matt felt a bit dizzy. He was having trouble catching his breath. He sat with his head down.

"Are you okay?" asked Matt's teammate Dave.

"I think so," answered Matt. "I'm just a little tired. I played almost the whole half. I'll be fine."

The coach told them all to tighten up their defense. "Stop playing sloppy," he said. "No more turnovers!"

They took the court to start the second half, but Matt did not feel better. As he took the tip-off down the court, the room seemed to spin. He fell to the floor.

Most Lyme carditis involves an arterial valve blockage, a blockage in a valve that allows blood to flow from the heart to the rest of the body. The restricted blood flow can cause lightheadedness, chest pain, or irregular heart rhythms. You may feel as if you are going to faint, especially after exercising.

Carditis can be caused by other conditions as well. Again, it will be important to tell your doctor of other symptoms you have experienced, even if they seem unrelated. Of course, if you have seen an EM rash, suspect Lyme disease.

Without the rash, a low-grade fever, fatigue, or general achiness can indicate a Lyme infection. Especially if there has been no previous evidence of heart disease and you are in good general health, you should probably speak to your doctor about testing for Lyme disease. Lyme carditis typically occurs three to five weeks after you have been infected.

Matt was rushed to the hospital where doctors tested his blood and his heart. They found an irregular heart rhythm. Further tests detected a blockage in Matt's aortal arterial heart valve. Dr. Burke met with Matt's parents, Laura and Sam.

"The valve in Matt's heart that lets blood flow through his aorta is blocked. There can be several causes for the blockage, so I would like to ask you a few questions."

"Anything," said Laura.

"In the spring and summer, does Matt spend a lot of time outdoors?" asked Dr. Burke.

"Yes, he loves to go fishing. There's a pond on the farm behind our house. He can get there by walking through the woods. On the weekends, I go with him," said Sam.

"This past summer, did you notice any strange rash on Matt? Did he have the flu or seem especially tired?"

"He didn't mention anything," said Laura. "He did seem to have the flu for a day or so, but he didn't have a high fever. And it went away quickly, so I didn't worry."

"I'll ask Matt about the rash," said Dr. Burke. "Matt's blood tested positive for Lyme antibodies. I think it's possible that his heart problems were caused

24

by Lyme disease. He could have been infected in the summer. Without treatment, the bacteria can move throughout the body. It could have affected different organs months after Matt was bitten by an infected tick. We'll begin giving Matt antibiotics. In most cases, the medication corrects the blockage."

Once treatment with antibiotics is begun, Lyme carditis can usually be corrected. In rare instances, severe blockages continue and in some instances have led to death. Patients with these severe valve blockages may be hospitalized to better allow doctors to monitor the patient's heart. By early 2000, no studies of Lyme carditis had been conducted so the best treatment was still unknown.

The Psychological
Aspects of Lyme Disease

Peggy Wilson tried to take Dr. Monroe's advice. She was careful when she lifted Carrie from her car seat. She never lifted anything heavy. Even so, her back hurt so much that she could hardly move.

The pain kept her up at night. Because she didn't sleep, she was tired all the time. One day her boss, Mr. Madison, called her into his office.

"Peggy, you've been working here since you graduated from high school and have always done a great job," Mr. Madison said. "In fact, I've always counted on you to keep this department running smoothly. As long as you were out there, I knew I didn't have to worry about meeting our deadlines.

"But things have changed. You don't seem to have your mind on your work. You're always biting someone's head off. Just this morning, you barked at Mary because she asked where you had put the Wendell-Holmes file. You said 'How should I know?' when the file was lying on top of your desk.

"The point is, Peggy," continued Mr. Madison. "I don't know how long I can put up with this. You've missed a lot of work lately. I'm putting you on a thirty-day probation. If you can't straighten up, I'm afraid I'll have to fire you."

"I don't know what's wrong with me," Peggy said. "My doctor tells me it's just stress. I'll try harder to get my work done."

Peggy went back to her desk. She really had no idea how she could try harder, but she had to say something to Mr. Madison. She wasn't being unkind on purpose. How could she just stop feeling tired and depressed and suddenly be her old cheerful self? I'm going to get fired, she thought. Then what will I do? I'll have no money and no health insurance. I'll never find out what's wrong with me.

When you have Lyme disease, in addition to dealing with physical symptoms, you may find yourself battling psychological difficulties. Especially if you are suffering with chronic Lyme disease, you may feel depressed and frustrated. Your disease may seem to have control over your life. Your academic, career, or athletic performance may be affected. Your friends may not understand your behavior and your social life may suffer. Sometimes, even though your parents are doing their best to help you, you may feel alone, like no one can understand what you are going through.

The ringing bell startled Jeremy awake. Oh no, he thought, I fell asleep again. Miss Waterman is going to have a fit.

Jeremy started to pick up his books. "Hey, man, you were totally out," said Jeremy's best friend, Eddie. "Waterman was giving you the evil eye. What's up anyway? How come you keep falling asleep?"

"I'm just tired," said Jeremy. He didn't want Eddie to know he was sick.

"Look out. Here comes Waterman," said Eddie. "I'm out of here."

Miss Waterman waited until the other students had left the room. "Jeremy, I need to talk to you," she said. "Please wait a minute. I'll give you a late pass to your next class."

"Okay," Jeremy said. He slumped down into his chair.

Miss Waterman sat in the desk next to Jeremy. "This is the third time this week that you have fallen asleep. It's not normal for you, Jeremy, so I think there must be something wrong outside of this class. Is there something that you want to tell me?"

"I don't know," said Jeremy.

"I'm not as scary as you may think," said Miss Waterman. "I'd like to help you if I can."

"I have Lyme disease," said Jeremy. "I have pain in my joints. Sometimes I feel it in my back or elbows. Sometimes my hands hurt so much that I can't hold a pencil. Usually my knees hurt. The pain keeps me awake at night, so I'm real tired during the day. I'm sorry I fell asleep again."

"I think you should have your parents set up a meeting with the guidance office," said Miss Waterman. "Your other teachers should understand that you're not just being lazy. But you may also want to call a therapist, someone you can talk to about how you feel."

"I don't need a therapist," said Jeremy. "I'm not crazy."

"That's exactly my point," said Miss Waterman. "You're not crazy. But just saying it probably doesn't make you feel better. You may feel a little crazy some of the time. Talking about how you feel with someone who doesn't judge you for it can be very helpful. They can help you understand and deal with the new feelings that you are having."

"I'll think about it," said Jeremy.

In reality, it will be difficult for other people to understand how you feel. You may want to find a support group in your area. If you live in an area where Lyme disease is common, you will probably be able to find a support group specifically for people with this disease. If there are no Lyme disease support groups, you may be able to find one for people suffering from chronic diseases. In a support group, you will find people like you who live each day with Lyme disease. They will understand and sympathize with your frustration. They will not think you are weird or that you are acting like a baby. They will not think you should "just get over it." Oftentimes, groups are sponsored by hospitals or led by therapists. Sometimes someone who suffers or has suffered from Lyme disease will be the group leader. You may be able to find information about support groups from your doctor or a nearby hospital. If not, Lyme disease organizations such as the Lyme Disease Network and the Lyme Alliance may be able to help you. (See the Where to Go for Help section at the back of this book for contact information.)

When Allie walked into Dr. Winkler's office, Dr. Winkler could see that she was depressed.

"How are you feeling, Allie?" asked Dr. Winkler.

"If I felt okay, I wouldn't need to come here," said Allie. "I'm sick of coming here. I'm sick of being sick. I'm tired all the time. I can't do anything. My life feels useless."

"It's not unusual to have those feelings," said Dr. Winkler. "You've been sick for a long time. Have you ever considered going to a support group?"

"What's that?" asked Allie.

"A support group is a group of people who share the same problem. Alcoholics Anonymous is a support group for people who are addicted to alcohol. There are also support groups for people with Lyme disease."

"What's the point of sitting around with a bunch of sick people?" asked Allie.

"Other people with Lyme disease will understand how you feel," answered Dr. Winkler. "You can talk to them. They may have some ideas that will help you deal with your disease."

"I don't want to talk to people I don't know," said Allie.

"You could try just listening for a while," suggested Dr. Winkler. "No one will force you to talk if you don't want to. Then when you feel comfortable with the members of the group, you may want to join the conversation."

"Where do I have to go for this group?" asked Allie.

"It meets at Union County Hospital. I have a brochure in my office with dates and times. I'll get it for you."

"Okay, maybe I'll try it," said Allie.

30

Keep in mind that support groups are not designed to treat people with serious clinical depression, although they can probably help with the feelings of unhappiness that usually accompany chronic illness. According to a Harvard Medical School study, if you are experiencing extreme fatigue, loss of appetite, sleeplessness, difficulty concentrating, or loss of memory, you may be suffering from major depression. In this case, you might be better off seeking private therapy while also continuing with your support group.

If you are suffering from Lyme disease, you may also feel guilty about the toll your illness is taking on your family. Your illness may cause a financial burden as well as physical and emotional frustration for your parents and siblings. You may also feel that you are letting down friends, coworkers, or teammates because you are unable to make yourself well.

In his junior year, Todd had been the quarterback of the football team at Western High. The team, called the Hawks, had won the county playoffs but had lost to St. Mary's in the first game of the states. After that game, Todd and his teammates had sworn on an oath to do everything possible to bring home the state trophy next year.

But suddenly everything went wrong. Todd became infected with Lyme disease. He had seen the EM rash but didn't know what it was. The rash went away, and Todd felt fine for a while.

But soon he began to feel dizzy. His legs ached. He worked out with the other football players in the gym, but the weight training became more and more painful. He finally went to the doctor. Todd had Lyme disease.

Todd's doctor had given him pills to take. He felt better for a while, but then his joints began to ache again. The intravenous antibiotics worked at first, too. But the pain always returned.

In the cafeteria at lunchtime, John, the center on the football team, started talking to Todd about the next season.

"I can't wait—man, we'll be great," said John. "St. Mary's quarterback graduated. So did that little pipsqueak running back. He was small but he sure could run. With those two gone, we should have no problem taking the trophy."

"I don't know if I'll be able to play," said Todd.

"What do you mean?" said John. "You have to play. We're nothing without you. Morrison's an okay backup, but he can't throw a bomb like you can. We'll never win without you."

"I can't help it," said Todd.

"Well, you better help it," John said. "The team's counting on you."

"But You Look Fine!"

Even though you may be dealing with chronic Lyme disease, you probably don't look sick. This can make it hard for people to believe that you have a serious illness. When an individual's disability or disease is obvious, others feel sympathy. But because Lyme disease is not always obvious, people who do not understand your illness may think that you are faking or exaggerating the severity of your symptoms. Others may think that you are just trying to get attention. This can add to your feelings of guilt and frustration.

Private Therapy

If you are experiencing severe depression or you have issues that are not being dealt with in your support group, you may want to consider seeking a private therapist. Ask the doctor treating your physical symptoms to suggest a psychologist, psychiatrist, or therapist who can help you with your emotional and psychological symptoms. A therapist should listen to you talk about your feelings and help you understand them. He or she should help you see that you are not to blame for your illness. And a therapist should be able to help you explain your condition to your friends so that they will understand, too.

When Melanie got home, she went straight to her room. She switched on the radio and turned up the volume. It didn't matter what the song was as long as it was loud. Melanie lay on the bed, staring up at the ceiling. Tears ran from her eyes and down the sides of her face.

Melanie was alone because her mom had needed to get a job. Her dad was a landscaper and because his business was small, his health insurance benefits were limited. Melanie's medical expenses were very high, and they were not always covered. To help pay the bills, her mom had begun working part-time as a waitress at the West Side Diner.

33

It's my fault she has to work, thought Melanie. If I hadn't gotten sick everything would be fine.

At school that day, some of the kids had teased her. "I went to the diner last night and guess who I saw," Brittany had said. "Your mom! She even waited on our table. But don't worry, my dad left a big tip. I told him you must really need the money."

Melanie had been embarrassed and ashamed. Now she was ashamed of feeling embarrassed. She hated that her mom was waitressing, especially where her friends could see her. But she also hated herself. Everything that has gone wrong is my fault, Melanie thought.

Illness can be isolating. Try not to cut yourself off from your parents and others who love you. Communicating openly about your feelings will help everyone in your family cope with Lyme disease.

Lyme Anxiety

The yard behind Jason's house was a long slope. In the winter, he and his friends spent hours sledding and snowboarding. Now, on this sunny spring day, the snow had melted. Jason and his friend Derrick looked sadly down the hill.

"I wish we could still snowboard," said Derrick. "I loved racing down the hill. I'm bored."

"Me, too," said Jason. "Wait a minute. Maybe we don't need snowboards. We could rake up those dead leaves and pile them at the bottom of the hill." He pointed to the leaves that had blown around the

bushes and shrubs. "Then we could lie down and roll down the hill into the leaves. What do you think?"

Jason and Derrick raked and piled the leaves. Then they took turns rolling down the hill and into the leaves. They had a great time. Jason's mom could hear them whooping and cheering as they rolled faster and faster.

At dinner time, Derrick headed home and Jason went into the house. "It sounded like you and Derrick were having a great time," said Jason's mom.

"It was great," said Jason. "Almost as good as snowboarding."

Suddenly, Jason's mom noticed a tick crawling up Jason's arm. "Hold on," she said. "That's a tick. They carry Lyme disease. I'm calling Dr. Wilson right away."

Jason's mom called the doctor and made an appointment for that same afternoon. Jason did not want to go.

"Come on, Mom. I feel fine," he said.

"You could have Lyme disease and still feel fine," she answered. "We're going to the doctor."

At Dr. Wilson's office, Jason's mom described the tick she had seen. Dr. Wilson listened carefully.

"I think Jason should start taking antibiotics, don't you?" said Jason's mom. "He could have Lyme disease and that can be very dangerous. We can't take any chances."

"You're right. Lyme disease can be dangerous," said Dr. Wilson. "But that doesn't mean everyone who sees a tick should start taking medicine. The tick you saw was not attached to Jason. He can't be infected with Lyme disease just from a crawling tick.

The tick must bite him to send the bacteria into his blood. Also, the tick you described was probably a dog tick. Dog ticks are bigger than deer ticks and easier to see. Deer ticks, especially in their early life stage, are so tiny you probably would not have casually noticed one until it had begun to enlarge. You have to look very carefully to find a young deer tick."

"But why should we wait?" asked Jason's mom. "Isn't it better to start the medication just in case? Better safe than sorry, I always say."

"Not necessarily," said Dr. Wilson. "Taking needless medication is not a good idea. In this case, the evidence of infection is not strong enough. You were right to be worried about the tick. We should all be concerned when we find ticks on our bodies. But I do not believe that Jason has Lyme disease. I don't think he should take antibiotics now. But if you see an EM rash, call me right away. Also, if Jason feels feverish or has joint or muscle pain, bring him right in. And keep checking for ticks."

"Thank you, Dr. Wilson," she said. "And Jason, no more rolling down the hill into dead leaves. Try riding your bike instead."

"Oh, Mom," said Jason.

The fear of Lyme disease can cause another form of psychological trauma called Lyme anxiety. In areas where Lyme disease is most prevalent, public information campaigns have increased awareness both in doctors and the general public. For the most part, this awareness has been beneficial. However, some people have become so concerned about Lyme disease that they regard any symptoms similar to those of Lyme disease as a sure sign that they have the disease. Sometimes, parents demand that their children be treated with antibiotics whenever they suspect the possibility of Lyme disease. For example, if they find an unattached tick crawling on their child and that child develops a fever, the parents may demand that their doctor begin antibiotics. Some doctors may prescribe antibiotics "just to be on the safe side." But generally, taking unnecessary medication is not a good idea.

The tick you find crawling on your leg could be a dog tick, which shares the deer tick's habitat but does not cause Lyme disease. If you find an attached tick, watch the bite area carefully and be on the lookout for unusual symptoms, but there is no need to jump to conclusions.

Difficulties of Diagnosis

"While we wait for the test results, I'm going to have you admitted to the hospital, Claire," said Dr. Connolly. "If the tests confirm that you have Lyme disease, and I think they will, you will need to begin intravenous antibiotic treatment right away."

After several hours, Dr. Connolly met with Claire and her parents. "The test results show that we were right—Claire has Lyme disease," she said. "Her blood already contains Lyme antibodies. The antibodies are trying to fight the bacteria that are causing her illness. We need to give those antibodies a boost, to help them fight.

"You'll need to stay in the hospital for a couple of days. When we know the antibiotics are working, you can go home and take pills to continue your treatment."

Lyme disease can sometimes be very hard to diagnose because it can be mistaken for so many other diseases. Especially if you do not get the EM rash, you may think that your early symptoms—headache, achiness, and fatigue— are caused by some other more common illness, like the flu. We also learned how Stage II and Stage III Lyme disease can be mistaken for other serious conditions. The joint pain of Lyme arthritis can be mistaken for rheumatoid arthritis. Symptoms that affect the brain and nervous system are sometimes confused with multiple sclerosis.

This possibility of misdiagnosis can work against you in two ways. First, the doctor may begin treatment for another illness, which he or she believes to be the cause of the symptoms. In this case, the Lyme disease may be left untreated and worsen. On the other hand, a doctor may begin treatment for Lyme disease when the symptoms are in fact caused by another disease. You may receive unnecessary treatment for Lyme disease while the true condition is left untreated.

If you are sick, you and your doctor will want to find the cause. Sometimes the best course seems to be to accept the first diagnosis. You finally have a name for what is causing your illness. You feel there is something you can do about it. You and your doctor are in control of your situation.

But if the diagnosis is inaccurate, accepting it can have dire consequences. Untreated Lyme disease can continue to spread throughout your body.

Obviously, careful diagnosis is important. But it is also critical to monitor the results of any treatment. If you do not feel a treatment is helping, discuss your concerns with your doctor. Keep a diary or log of your symptoms and how they are affected by treatment. It may help your doctor prescribe the correct medication.

According to the Centers for Disease Control and Prevention (CDC), in addition to checking your physical symptoms, your doctor should ask you some important questions to find out if you were exposed to ticks.

⮩ Do you live in, or were you visiting, an area where deer ticks are common?

➥ Have you recently spent time outdoors, especially in wooded areas or places with tall grass?

➥ Do you go hiking, fishing, or hunting?

➥ Do you play outdoor spring or summer sports, such as soccer, basketball, softball, or field hockey?

➥ Do you remember finding a tick attached to your body?

You need to answer all of the questions your doctor asks as completely as possible. Remember, you could have been bitten by a tick weeks or even months before you experience any symptoms. You will need to think very carefully to help your doctor make the correct diagnosis. The more information you can give your doctor, the easier if will be for him or her to properly diagnose your condition.

There are also blood tests to help doctors diagnose Lyme disease. These tests are not always accurate, though, especially if you are in the first stage of Lyme disease. Up to a month after you are bitten by an infected tick, the most common test, called an ELISA titer, may not show a positive result, even if you are infected. This is because the test does not check for the Lyme disease bacteria. Instead, it looks for antibodies, the defensive cells that your body makes to fight off the disease. If you were only recently infected, your body may not yet have made enough antibodies for the test to detect them. Another test, the Western blot test, also looks for Lyme antibodies. But according to the instructions laid down by the CDC, only patients who test positive on the ELISA titer should be given the Western blot test as a confirmation. Patients who test negative on the ELISA test, according to the CDC, do not need to be given the Western blot test.

According to the International Lyme and Associated Diseases Society (ILADS), some doctors believe that the Western blot is the most effective test. However, if the CDC guidelines are followed, patients whose blood tests negative on the ELISA titer may never receive the Western blot. Studies have shown that the ELISA titer can fail to accurately diagnose Lyme disease more that 50 percent of the time. The National Institutes of Health now supports several research projects to develop new tests that will be more accurate and reliable.

Sometimes tests are fooled because they don't accurately differentiate between Lyme antibodies and antibodies for other diseases. You may test positive for Lyme disease when your symptoms are really caused by something else. Also, people who have been vaccinated for Lyme disease will test positive for the disease.

Researchers are working on a new test that has proven more accurate when used to detect the disease at the early stages of infection. Currently, tests detect antibodies that are loose and unattached to the Lyme disease bacteria. These unbound antibodies are often not present in large enough numbers in the earliest stages of infection. The new test finds antibodies that are attached to the surface of Lyme bacteria. These bound antibodies form in the very early stages of the disease. In studies by the University of Dentistry and Medicine in New Jersey, 96 percent of patients with active Lyme disease tested positive using the new test. During early 2000, follow-up studies were still being conducted. Researchers expected that the new test would be available sometime during 2001.

While doctors use some tests to find Lyme disease, other tests are used to rule out other illnesses. These tests do not prove that you have Lyme disease, but they rule out other illnesses that have similar symptoms. They help determine that your illness, especially the more severe symptoms of disseminated or chronic Lyme disease, is not caused by a different problem. Some of these tests are:

- Electroencephalogram (EEG)—An EEG measures electrical activity in your brain. Abnormal activity can cause seizure disorders. A normal EEG helps to rule out brain abnormalities.

- Magnetic resonance imaging (MRI)—With the help of computer analysis, an MRI uses a magnetic field to look inside your body. Detailed images help doctors find tumors. Doctors can also use the computer generated "pictures" to find areas of your body that may be damaged or diseased.

- Computerized axial tomography (CAT scan)— During a CAT scan, dozens of X-ray "pictures" are taken of the inside of your body. Usually, a CAT scan is directed at a specific part, like your brain. A computer links these pictures to give doctors more information and help them make a diagnosis.

↪ Visual evoked responses (VER)—The VER is used to rule out multiple sclerosis.

↪ Spinal tap—To perform a spinal tap, or lumbar puncture, your doctor will use a long needle to extract a small amount of the fluid that surrounds your spinal cord. This test would probably be used only if your CNS has been affected. An analysis of the spinal fluid will help doctors find evidence of other infections.

According to the Lyme Disease Foundation, no test can rule out Lyme disease. All available tests are designed to help doctors determine whether you have Lyme disease. But no test proves that you do not have Lyme disease. The most important information will come from you. Understanding Lyme disease and its symptoms may be your best defense.

Kelly Watson had been sick for four years, since she was twelve years old. She lived in a wooded area of Massachusetts and frequently saw deer in her backyard. But Kelly rarely felt like spending time outdoors. She was very tired most of the time. She had headaches that seemed to move around inside her head. Sometimes she felt dizzy or nauseous. Since she was twelve, her knees, ankles, wrists, and even her hands hurt. Her back ached. Today, Kelly and her mom were on the way to a doctor's office, a trip that had become very familiar to Kelly.

Kelly's mom had taken her to the doctor four years ago. She told the doctor that as far as she knew, Kelly had not been bitten by a tick. Neither Kelly nor her mom remembered seeing an EM rash. Although Kelly's joints were painful, they were not swollen.

The doctor had taken blood to perform several tests. One laboratory reported that Kelly's tests did not show Lyme disease. Other lab tests reported a positive result.

Kelly's doctor had diagnosed Lyme disease and begun treatment with antibiotics. First, Kelly took pills for four months, but she did not get better. The doctor tried intravenous antibiotics. The drugs caused problems in Kelly's intestines and did not help her other symptoms.

Over the next three years, Kelly's symptoms had improved a bit and then worsened again. The doctor had tried other drugs. One caused more digestive problems. Another gave Kelly hives.

Mrs. Watson had decided to try another doctor. Now they were headed to see Dr. Ellis, a specialist in infectious diseases. Earlier, all of Kelly's files had been sent to Dr. Ellis to give him a chance to review them before seeing her.

After examining Kelly, Dr. Ellis asked her and Mrs. Watson to join him in his consultation room.

"I've gone over all of Kelly's tests and the results of her past treatments," said Dr. Ellis. "Her most recent blood test shows a negative result for Lyme disease. She has not responded to antibiotic therapy and in fact has suffered some very serious side effects. Neither of you can remember a tick bite or an EM rash. All of these facts suggest that Kelly does not have Lyme disease and that her symptoms are caused by another disorder.

"I'm particularly concerned about the length of time you spend sleeping, Kelly," continued Dr. Ellis. "Tell me again, please, how many hours you sleep in a day."

"I'm always exhausted when I get home from school," Kelly said. "So I need to take a nap."

"How long do your naps usually last?" asked Dr. Ellis.

"Usually about three hours. Once I was still asleep when Mom came home from work at 6:30," answered Kelly.

"That's a very long nap. When do you usually go to bed and wake up?" Dr. Ellis asked.

"I go to bed around 10:00 PM. I have to get up for school at 7:10 AM."

"Do you still feel tired in the morning?"

"Usually," said Kelly.

"I'm sure that you're sick of doctors," said Dr. Ellis. "But I'm afraid I have to recommend that you see another one. I'm sending you to Dr. Winslow. She has a lot of experience dealing with a condition called fibromyalgia. Fibromyalgia causes joint pain that is seemingly unexplained. It can also cause burning feelings and numbness. Fatigue is another symptom. For some reason, women seem to suffer from fibromyalgia more often than men."

"You're right, Dr. Ellis," said Mrs. Watson. "We are sick of doctors. But we are more sick of Kelly's pain. If Dr. Winslow will be able to help Kelly, we'll be glad to see her."

Treating Lyme Disease

Mr. Melton made an appointment with Dr. Canning for the next afternoon.

"So, I hear you have a 'really weird' rash, Nathan," said Dr. Canning. "Can I see it please?"

Nathan lifted his arm. Dr. Canning examined the rash, running his fingers over Nathan's skin.

"Does it hurt when I touch it?" asked Dr. Canning.

"No," said Nathan.

"If you didn't live in a city, I would be sure this rash is a symptom of Lyme disease," said Dr. Canning. "But we don't find many ticks here. Have you been away on vacation recently?"

"Yes, I was visiting my relatives at the shore last week," said Nathan. "I'm an amateur photographer and I especially like to take pictures of wildlife. I also walked their dog, Elsie. She's a black lab."

"You probably picked up a deer tick and it bit you. Some ticks are so tiny that it is very difficult to see them. A tick bite does not hurt so it's not surprising that you didn't notice it.

"I'll give you a prescription for amoxicillin, an antibiotic. The antibiotic will help your body's natural defenses fight the disease. Because you found the rash early and will begin treatment right away, you

should be fine. But if you still get headaches or feel like you have the flu, call me right away."
"We will," said Mr. Melton.

Early Treatment

According to the American Lyme Disease Foundation, if you begin treatment within three to six weeks of the day you were infected, Lyme disease is almost always easily cured. Most likely, your doctor will prescribe antibiotics for you to take. Stage I Lyme disease can usually be treated successfully with fourteen to twenty-eight days of oral antibiotics in pill form, usually amoxicillin. The key to a cure, the complete elimination of all Lyme disease symptoms, is early treatment, before the disease reaches Stage II, or disseminated, Lyme disease.

Treating Disseminated Lyme Disease

Disseminated Lyme disease, like Lyme arthritis, is more difficult to treat. Your doctor may decide to intravenously (with an IV) administer the antibiotics through a needle directly into your bloodstream. This course of treatment—IV antibiotics—may require a hospital stay.

The doctor may decide to insert a catheter, a needle and tube, into your forearm to allow the medication to be directly pumped into your bloodstream. Because the catheter can stay in your arm for two to six weeks without being replaced, you will not need to remain in the hospital for this treatment. Most likely, you will need visits from a home health care agency.

Hidden Bacteria

If your symptoms were not diagnosed early, the bacteria may have had a chance to disperse inside your body and "hide." These hidden bacteria may not respond to an initial treatment of antibiotics. The bacteria can lie dormant, as if they were asleep, for months, and then "wake up." You may feel that your Lyme disease had been cured but then it returns.

During the course of your treatment, your doctor should probably give you periodic tests to determine the need to continue your medication. The doctor will also probably look for side effects such as a change in white blood cells or liver function. Long-term antibiotic therapy is controversial. Some doctors worry about the effects of chemical antibiotics on your body's natural immune system. They believe that antibiotics may cause the natural immune system to stop working properly. Other doctors use the example of tuberculosis treatment, where long-term antibiotics were used successfully, as evidence to support this treatment for Lyme disease. Doctors and scientists continue to study the best way to treat disseminated Lyme disease.

In any case, during your treatment you and your doctor must work closely together. You must be honest with your doctor and talk openly about your symptoms. Your doctor should listen and monitor your condition closely. Because the symptoms of Stage II and III Lyme disease are so variable, treatment can be difficult. The most important information your doctor receives will come from you. If you do not feel that your doctor understands your symptoms or listens respectfully to you, consider finding a new doctor.

Dangerous Treatments

Some people who have not found a satisfactory cure for their Lyme disease have become desperate and looked outside of conventional medicine for treatment. One such treatment involves injecting a diluted solution of hydrogen peroxide into the bloodstream in the hope that the chemical will kill the Lyme bacteria. This procedure is dangerous and does not work.

Another treatment is based on the theory that the Lyme bacteria cannot live in high heat. Patients travel to Mexico to have themselves deliberately infected with malaria, a disease that causes high fever. The patients believe that the high body temperature during the malaria fever will kill the Lyme bacteria. Malaria is another painful, dangerous, and potentially lingering disease. No one should contract it on purpose. This treatment has not been proven to cure Lyme disease.

You should also beware of treatments that seem too good to be true or do not make sense. Treatments that promise a quick cure should be questioned. Meditation or herbal therapies may help relieve symptoms but should not be used as a replacement for a doctor's care.

Physical Therapy and Exercise

Physical therapy has proven to be helpful, especially for patients suffering with arthritis or physical weakness. Talk to your doctor about your plans to begin an exercise program. Begin slowly. Your doctor may recommend a physical therapist to guide your progress.

49

Treatment Resistant Lyme Disease

During his senior year in high school, Greg was the star pitcher on his baseball team. That year his team had a record of fifteen wins and only two losses. They made it to the semifinals of the state championships.

That was only three years ago, but it seemed like a lifetime to Greg. His Lyme arthritis now kept him off the mound. The pain in his shoulder and knees prevented him from participating in any athletic activity.

Greg's Lyme disease was diagnosed about six months after he was first infected. His shoulders, elbows, hips, knees, fingers, and wrists were all affected. The pain moved from one joint to another, sometimes affecting several at the same time.

During his examination, Greg's doctor had talked to him about the symptoms of Lyme disease. Greg remembered seeing an EM rash in his armpit. The rash had lasted about two weeks. But it was never painful and Greg had not had any other symptoms until the arthritis began six months later.

First, Greg was given an oral antibiotic. When his knees remained swollen, he received a different antibiotic, this time intravenously.

Nearly two years after treatment began, Greg's blood tests still showed a high level of Lyme antibodies in his system, indicating that the bacteria was still present and his body was fighting hard against it. His doctors decided against continued treatment with antibiotics. Instead, they began treatments with steroids to reduce the inflammation in Greg's knees.

50

*Now, years after his Lyme disease was first diag-
nosed, Greg's knees are no longer swollen. Greg is
beginning to gain hope that he will be able to play
baseball again.*

In a small percentage of cases, the arthritis caused by
Lyme disease does not respond to antibiotics given either
in pill form or intravenously. Researchers are not sure why
this happens. One theory, which we talked about earlier,
suggests that the Lyme bacteria are able to hide, or
sequester, inside your body. The antibiotics do not find
these hidden bacteria and they can continue to make you
sick. Another theory suggests that some Lyme bacteria are
able to develop immunity, or resistance, to the antibiotics.
These Lyme bacteria are able to resist the medication and
your Lyme symptoms continue.

The mysteries of long-term Lyme disease continue to
perplex the medical community. Some people continue to
suffer from symptoms seemingly related to the disease for
years, while their doctors try everything they know to help
them. Doctors also continue testing various new treatments and work to better understand this painful and
debilitating disease in the hopes that they will soon find
an effective treatment.

The Habits and Habitats of Ticks

What are ticks? Scientists classify ticks as arachnids, like spiders. Ticks are not insects because they have three body segments (insects have two). Also, adult ticks have eight legs while insects have six. Ticks do not have wings or antennae, like insects.

Ticks are parasites. They live off the blood of another animal or a person, called the host. They cannot survive alone and depend on their hosts for food and to reproduce.

There are over 850 species of ticks in the world. In North America, five species of ticks can transmit disease to humans. The blacklegged tick, sometimes called the deer or bear tick, transmits Lyme disease bacteria from eastern North America through the Midwest. Along the Pacific coast and in northwestern states, the disease is transmitted by the Western blacklegged tick. The Northeast habitat is shared by the dog tick, which is considerably larger and does not transmit Lyme disease.

The Life Cycle of a Tick

In Connecticut, a white-tailed deer walked through the forest. She brushed against shrubs and tall grass. Sometimes she pulled leaves from the lower branches of young trees. At the edge of the woods, where the sunlight reached the ground, she lowered her head to graze.

The deer was unaware of the ticks that were crawling up her legs. Another tick was making its way down her neck to her shoulders. There it would burrow under her fur and bite.

The deer is infected with Lyme disease bacteria. Soon, the tick will be infected, too. The deer is not sick. She just carries the bacteria and passes them along to ticks that bite her. The ticks will pass the bacteria to other animals, like deer, mice, chipmunks, and other small animals that will carry the bacteria in their blood but will not become sick.

But other creatures become very sick when infected with Lyme bacteria. Dogs, horses, and humans suffer serious symptoms.

The tick does not intentionally infect other animals with Lyme bacteria. It is simply looking for a meal.

The two-year life cycle of a tick includes four stages. In each stage, the tick molts, or sheds, its old skeleton and grows a new one to fit its new body structure.

⇒ Egg—In the fall and early spring, adult ticks mate on large animals, like white-tailed deer. The female needs to feed in order to produce eggs, then drops off the deer to lay the eggs on the ground. The eggs hatch into larvae by summer.

⇒ Larvae—Sometimes called seed ticks, larvae have six legs and are very tiny. After they are hatched, they feed for about two days on mice and other small mammals. That meal will be enough to last them until the next spring when they will feed and molt into nymphs.

➣ Nymph—At this stage, the tick has all eight of its legs. It is now the size of a poppy seed or the period at the end of this sentence. Nymphs feed for about four days in the late spring and summer and molt into adults in the fall. You are most likely to get Lyme disease from a nymph because nymphs are the most active in spring and summer. They are also very hard to see because they are so tiny.

➣ Adult—In this final stage, the tick is the size of a sesame seed. When the female feeds, it swells up, or becomes engorged, until it is about the size of a pea.

Ticks can become infected with Lyme disease bacteria during the last three life stages. They carry the bacteria with them when they molt, infecting more mice, deer, and people when they feed.

A Tick's Home

Ticks like shady, moist areas. They are most often found near the ground, in dead leaves or low weeds. They can also cling to tall grass and shrubs up to three feet from the ground. But they cannot fly and they will not jump from a higher perch onto you. You must come into direct contact with them. From its perch on a leaf or twig, the tick waves its front legs in the air, behavior that researchers call "questing." It uses scent to detect when a host is nearby. It can also find a host by sensing body heat. Claws and adhesive pads at the tips of its legs help it latch on. Most likely, after reaching your skin, the tick will crawl upward to a more hidden spot, like the back of your knee or your armpit.

If ticks could choose their hosts, they would not choose you. They much prefer deer or mice. But they will take advantage of any opportunity to hitch a ride for a meal. If the opportunity arises, ticks will feed on raccoons, chipmunks, dogs, cats, or cattle. In fact, scientists have identified forty-nine species of birds and twenty-nine species of mammals, including humans, that can serve as tick hosts. Scientists believe that one of the reasons that Lyme disease is spreading so quickly is that so many animals can host ticks and therefore carry them from one place to another.

Lyme Disease "Hot Spots"

According to the CDC, you are most likely to get Lyme disease in the Northeast. New York, New Jersey, Pennsylvania, and Connecticut all reported more than 2,000 cases in 1997. However, it is south-central Connecticut, Westchester County and eastern Long Island in New York, the southern coast of New Jersey, and Cape Cod and Nantucket Island in Massachusetts that are considered the hyperendemic areas, or "hot spots." Other high incidence states include California, Minnesota, and Wisconsin. Connecticut's incident rate, 70.23 (the number of cases per 100,000 people), is more than double nearly every other state's. In 1997, Montana was the only state with no federally reported cases.

You should keep in mind, however, that these figures reflect only those cases reported to the CDC. In Connecticut, doctors are very aware of the symptoms of Lyme disease and are more likely to report it. Because the symptoms can resemble those of other illnesses, Lyme disease is suspected to be misreported, especially in states where the incidence is low. Because doctors in these areas are not as familiar with the disease, they sometimes do not recognize it. Other times, doctors may confuse a patient's symptoms and diagnose Lyme disease when the symptoms are actually caused by another kind of infection. Some doctors just do not bother to report Lyme disease when they have diagnosed it.

You do not need to live in a high-risk area to be infected. If you plan to vacation in the woods of Wisconsin or at the beaches of Cape Cod, Massachusetts, be careful. Not only can you become infected while on vacation, you can bring ticks home with you on your clothing or in camping gear.

Research has shown that ticks can hitch a ride not only on you, but also on migrating birds. That means ticks can come to you, wherever you live. A recent study by the British Columbia Center for Disease Control Society (BCCDCS) in Canada shows that songbirds may carry ticks. The birds fly through the mid-Atlantic and New England states during their spring migration, stopping to feed and rest on the way. When they fly on to their breeding areas in Canada, they may be carrying hitchhiking ticks. The BCCDCS found ticks infected with Lyme bacteria in Nova

56

Scotia, Prince Edward Island, New Brunswick, Quebec, Ontario, and Manitoba. It makes sense that if birds carry ticks north, birds can carry ticks south as well.

You can be bitten at any time of year, but the peak season is April to September in the Northeast and November to April on the West Coast. If an infected tick bites you, you can get Lyme disease even if you have already had it.

The incidence of Lyme disease is higher in the Northeast because large numbers of deer and white-footed mice live there. These animals have adapted to live successfully near humans. Ticks need deer and mice to survive and reproduce. Mice and deer carry the bacteria in their bloodstreams and infect ticks, but they do not get sick. When an infected tick bites you, the bacteria enter your bloodstream. Those bacteria can be carried all through your body.

Becoming Infected: How Do You Get Lyme Disease?

The answer to how you get Lyme disease is relatively simple. If you are bitten by an infected tick and do not remove it within forty-eight hours, you will probably become infected, too. Ticks do not actually cause the disease. They carry the bacteria and infect unsuspecting hosts by biting them. One of those hosts could be you. Now that you know where you might encounter ticks, you can be on the lookout for them if you live in those areas or visit them on your vacation. (See chapter 7 for information about safely removing ticks.)

Protecting Yourself from Ticks

Christopher was heading out to meet Eric and Louis at West Ridge Park. They planned to go for a hike. Christopher was wearing his favorite shorts and T-shirt. He pulled on heavy socks and his hiking boots. He stopped at the refrigerator to fill his back-pack with granola bars, apples, and three bags of chips. He filled a bottle with water and put that in his pack, too. Just as he was leaving, his mom walked in to the kitchen.

"Wait a minute," said Jenny. "You can't go hiking in a T-shirt and shorts. You could easily pick up a tick. Please change into long pants and a long sleeved shirt."

"Come on, Mom. It's really hot. I'll die," said Christopher. "I have on my boots. Ticks can't fly, you know. They won't be able to get over my boots."

"I know ticks can't fly. But they can cling to tall grass or weeds that are higher than the top of your socks. They could also attach to your socks and then crawl up until they reach your skin. Put on your jeans, please. And tuck them into your socks.

"But I'll compromise a bit on the shirt," Jenny con-tinued. "Take your denim shirt with you. You don't have to wear it as long as you stay on the path. But if you go off the path, put on the shirt. It will help

protect you. I know you think I am being overprotective, but getting Lyme disease is much worse than being too hot. Do we have a deal?"

"Okay, I guess," said Christopher. "But what about Eric and Louis? I bet they wear shorts and T-shirts."

"I'm not their mother," said Jenny. "I know you've heard that before, but it's still true. I can't worry about the whole world. It's just your luck that you're the one I get to worry about."

"Great," said Christopher sarcastically as he went back to his room to change his clothes.

The best way to protect yourself from Lyme disease is to stay out of the woods, avoid tall grassy areas, never sit on the grass, walk around piles of dead leaves—in other words, stay indoors. But most of us would rather not spend a sunny summer day gazing out the window. Chances are, you enjoy hiking, gardening, camping, fishing, or some other outdoor activities. Especially if you live in or take vacations in areas that are the prime habitats for deer ticks, the American Lyme Disease Foundation suggests that you take these precautions when you could be exposed:

- Wear light-colored clothing made with a tight weave. You will be able to spot ticks more easily on light-colored cloth, and they will have trouble getting to your skin.

- Always wear enclosed shoes or boots. Save your sandals for the beach.

➴ Wear long pants tucked into your socks and a long-sleeved shirt tucked into your pants.

➴ Before you head into the woods, you may want to spray your clothes with insect repellent containing DEET. Other insect repellents also work against ticks. However, you should spray these products on your clothes before you put them on, and let them dry for at least two hours before you wear them. Karen Vanderhoof-Forschner, founder of the Lyme Disease Foundation, finds Avon's Skin-So-Soft Bath Oil to be a very effective mosquito, flea, and deer tick repellent. She believes that it is especially good for children and pregnant women because it is an all-natural blend that is not toxic.

➴ Wear a hat. Keep long hair pulled back so it does not swing loosely against bushes or tall grass.

➴ When gardening, pruning, or picking up dead leaves, wear light-colored gloves and check them frequently for ticks.

➴ Avoid sitting on the ground or on stone walls where small animals like mice and chipmunks, which often carry ticks, may hide. Ticks looking for a meal from a mouse may find you instead. When you are attending an outdoor concert or picnicking where you must sit on the ground, use a blanket that has been sprayed with the same insect repellent you use on your clothing. If possible, bring lawn chairs.

↩ When hiking, stay on cleared, well-traveled paths whenever possible.

↩ While you are out in the woods or working in your garden, check yourself and others for ticks every three or four hours. Don't give ticks a chance to climb under your clothes.

↩ When you get home from your hike or your fishing trip, change your clothes right away. It's best to remove your outer layer of clothes away from the living area of your house, like in the basement or garage. Check the clothes for ticks and wash them as soon as possible.

↩ Take a shower and wash your hair, checking your entire body for ticks, as soon as you get home. They like to crawl into places where it will be hard to find them. Look behind your knees, in your navel, behind your ears, at the nape of your neck, in your armpits—everywhere! Pay special attention to areas where underwear elastic or bands from pants and shirts touch your skin. Use a hand-held mirror to inspect hard-to-see places.

You need to be concerned about ticks even in cooler weather. Ticks are active when the temperature is above forty degrees Fahrenheit. A complete self-examination whenever you have been outside in wooded or grassy areas is your best protection against infection.

Protecting Your Home

Linda and Dan Peterson were hard at work in their yard. They lived next door to the Liptons and had heard about Claire's Lyme disease.

"Lyme disease can be really scary," said Linda. "I wouldn't want Lydia to get bitten by a tick. She's so small."

"We're going to do everything we can to make sure none of us gets Lyme disease," said Dan. "Cleaning up our yard will help to keep ticks as far away from us as possible."

"Good idea," said Linda. "We should cut back the weeds and high grass on both sides of the fence."

"We can rake up all those dead leaves that got stuck under the bushes," said Dan. "Damp, cool places like that are perfect breeding grounds for ticks. I'll prune back these shrubs, too. And let's take down that bird feeder. We can hang it again in the winter, but I think the birds will do fine on their own for the summer."

"Okay. I'll get the rakes and we can get started," said Linda.

"Be sure to bring the work gloves," said Ed. "We don't want to get bitten by ticks while we're cleaning up the yard to get rid of them!"

In addition to protecting your body, you can also reduce the risk of exposure to ticks around your house. Keep the lawns mowed. Ticks prefer moist areas and tall grass. Clear brush and leaf litter away from the house, gardens, or stone walls.

62

Stack woodpiles neatly in a dry location, preferably off the ground. Mice often make nests in woodpiles. Be sure to wear gloves and a shirt with long sleeves when carrying firewood into the house.

Clean gardens of dead leaves and dried perennials in the fall when ticks are less active. If you wait until spring, choose a cool day when the temperature is below forty degrees. It may be more fun to garden on a warm, sunny spring day. But ticks are coming out to enjoy that sunshine, too.

Try not to invite animals that may be carrying ticks into your yard. Bird feeders do not only welcome cardinals and finches. The seeds that fall to the ground attract mice, chipmunks, and squirrels. If you have a bird feeder, keep the ground under it clean. Feed birds only in winter, when the risk of tick contamination is low.

Do not provide salt licks or food for deer. A fence can keep deer and the ticks they carry away from your home.

Scientists are working to keep deer away from residential areas and to reduce the tick population at the same time. A Yale University study funded by the United States Department of Agriculture is investigating the effectiveness of a four-poster deer feeder. Specially constructed feeding stations attract deer away from shrubs or gardens near homes. As the deer feeds at the station, insecticide is applied directly to its body.

Chemical Protection

Chemical insecticides may also be applied to lawns to control ticks. As with the use of any chemical, risks come with the benefits. Be sure to read the warnings on the product labels carefully and take any necessary precautions. Also, if your neighbors do not spray their lawns, too, ticks from next door will probably repopulate on your property. The Lyme Disease Coalition of New Jersey offers these recommendations for chemically controlling ticks:

↪ May 1–15—Granular diazinon or sevin (carbaryl) against nymphs.

↪ July 31—Damminix against larvae and nymphs will help control ticks and the infection rate for the next year.

↪ August 1–21—Repeat the May application.

↪November 1–20—Liquid permethrin or liquid/ granular diazinon or sevin against adult ticks.

If you use liquid sprays, apply them after 10:00 AM to expose the most questing ticks. Do not spray on windy days. Be sure to check all warnings and precautions when considering using chemical insecticides.

Removing Ticks Safely

If you are bitten by a tick, and you find it still on your skin, there are specific means that should be taken to remove the tick. If you remove the tick improperly, the area can become infected and may require a doctor visit.

When Christopher, Eric, and Louis met up at West Ridge Park, they decided to hike to a cave they had discovered near the top of the ridge. The entrance to the cave had been covered by the limbs of a fallen tree. They had to crawl under the tree to get inside the cool, dark cave. They kept the entrance covered, piling more dead branches over it. They were sure that no one else knew about the cave. It was their secret place.

That night, Christopher felt really tired. He decided to go to bed earlier than usual. While he was drying off after his shower, he noticed a tiny black speck in his armpit. He tried to brush the speck away, but it was stuck to his skin. He got partly dressed, then went to find his mom.

"Mom, can you look at this thing?" he said.

"Look at what 'thing'?" she asked.

"I have this really weird black bump in my armpit. I can't see it very well. What is it?"

"That's a tick," Jenny said. "Did you even wear your denim shirt?"

"No. And this is gross!" said Christopher.

"Yes, ticks are pretty gross," said Jenny. "They don't serve any useful purpose that I know of. Now, hold still."

Using tweezers, she carefully held the tick as close to Christopher's skin as possible and pulled firmly. Then after she washed her hands, she put antiseptic on the bite wound.

"You need to keep a close eye on the spot to be sure you don't get a 'bull's eye' rash, a rash that looks like red rings surrounding the place where the tick *was attached," she said. "If you see one, tell me right away. The rash will mean that you have Lyme disease and we'll need to get you checked by a doctor. You should probably call Eric and Louis so they can check for ticks, too."*

"Gross," Christopher said again.

Even if a tick has gotten a hold on your skin, you may have time to remove it before it can infect you with Lyme disease. Removing a tick within thirty-six hours after it becomes attached will greatly reduce your risk of becoming infected.

To remove that tick, use fine-tipped tweezers, grasp the tick's head, as close to the skin as possible. Do not hold the tick by the body. You want to remove the mouthparts from under your skin, if possible. Firmly and steadily, pull straight back, away from the skin. After you have removed the tick, wipe the bite area with disinfectant. Put the tick in a vial, if you plan to have it tested for disease, or in a jar of alcohol to kill it. You can also wrap it in a small piece of toilet paper and flush it down the toilet. Do not squash the tick, especially if it has become engorged, because you may release infected blood. Even though you have not handled the tick with your bare hands, be sure to wash them immediately after disposing of the tick.

Christopher often checked the spot where he had removed the tick. He did not get a red, spreading rash. He felt fine. "I don't think you have Lyme disease," Jenny said. "Just be sure to let me know if your knees hurt. And next time you go hiking, you will wear all the protective clothing."

You may have heard people say that you should not try to pull off a tick. But many times this is the only effective, though sometimes risky, method of removal. Some people suggest that you cover the tick with petroleum jelly to smother it. But ticks need very little oxygen to live and by the time an infected tick is out of air, you will already be infected. Another suggestion is to hold a hot match against the tick to make it release its hold and back out. But remember, ticks are tiny! You are much more likely to burn yourself than to make a tick move using this method.

Testing the Tick

Just to be on the safe side, Jenny decided to have the tick tested. She already had a small plastic container and information from a nearby lab. Lyme disease was very common in her area. She had read that this lab was conducting a study of ticks and Lyme disease. The lab tested ticks at no charge. Last month, Jenny had visited the lab and picked up the instructions for submitting ticks for testing. She wanted to be prepared.

Jenny put the tick in the plastic container and sealed it. She would drop it off at the lab during her lunch hour tomorrow.

Once you have removed the tick, you may want to have it tested to see if it is infected with Lyme disease.

But do not depend on this test to determine whether you have Lyme disease. Keep looking for the EM rash at the bite spot and monitor your health. If you feel Lyme disease symptoms, see your doctor right away.

Your local health department may do tick testing. If not, you can mail the tick to a test center. Before you send the tick, contact the test center to find out procedures, prices, and response time.

Lyme Disease in Animals

Animals can get Lyme disease, too. Dogs, cats, and horses can all become very sick when bitten by an infected tick. How can you protect your pet from infection? First and most important, remember that you are your pet's best defense against Lyme disease. Your pets cannot protect themselves.

Dogs and Cats

Nathan spent Labor Day weekend visiting his relatives at the Jersey shore again. He arrived Friday afternoon and expected a big, bouncy greeting from Elsie, their Labrador retriever. But Elsie did not jump up to greet him. Nathan thought Elsie looked sad.

Nathan called Elsie. "Come on, Elsie." But when she tried to get up, she fell down again. She wagged he tail weakly.

"Aunt Mona," Nathan called. "What's up with Elsie? I don't think she can walk!"

Mona leaned over to Elsie. "Come on, girl," she said gently. But Elsie just wagged her tail again. She could not get up.

"We better get Uncle Fred and take Elsie to the vet," said Mona. "I think that she may have Lyme disease. Our friend Mary's collie, Gretchen, had it last

69

year. Gretchen was okay after the vet gave Mary some pills to give her."

While Mona called the vet, Nathan helped his uncle carry Elsie to the car. When they got to the office, the receptionist asked them about Elsie's symptoms.

"She was fine yesterday," said Fred. "But today she was walking a bit stiff-legged. By the time Nate got here today, the poor girl couldn't walk at all. You know something's wrong when she doesn't jump up to say hi to Nate. She usually goes nuts when she sees him."

"She probably has Lyme disease," said the receptionist. "We see a lot of that this time of year. But don't worry. Dogs recover better than people."

"I hope so," said Fred.

"Me, too," said Nathan.

For several reasons, your dog is much more likely to become infected with Lyme disease than you are. Dogs need to spend time outdoors. Unleashed dogs pay no attention to paths, choosing instead to follow their noses, even if it takes them crashing through the underbrush. Fur provides an easy way for ticks to latch on to them. As wagging tails sweep through the grass, they pick up ticks. Ticks are hard to see against a dog's fur, especially when it is a dark color.

When should you suspect that your dog has been infected? Sometimes it is hard to tell. Your dog may seem listless, less energetic than usual, and sleep most of the time. He or she may have a fever or eat less. The most dramatic symptoms are similar to arthritis. If you know that your dog has not suffered any injury but seems to be having difficulty walking, you should probably ask your vet to test him or her for Lyme disease. This is especially true if you live in one of the geographical areas where Lyme disease is common. Early detection and treatment with antibiotics usually results in a speedy and complete recovery.

"You can bring Elsie in here," said the receptionist. "Dr. Riley will be right in."

Nathan and his uncle carried Elsie to the examining room and made her comfortable on the table.

"What's the matter, Elsie?" asked Dr. Riley as he walked into the room.

"We think maybe she has Lyme disease," said Uncle Fred.

"Did you find any ticks on her?" asked Dr. Riley.

"We find 'em and we just pull 'em off. She's never been sick before," said Uncle Fred.

"Most of the time, you were probably finding dog ticks. They're bigger and they don't carry Lyme disease. But it looks like a deer tick got her this time," said Dr. Riley. "She hasn't had any injuries lately, has she?"

"Nope," said Uncle Fred. "She spends a lot of time sleeping."

"I'm going to do some tests just to be sure that her nerves aren't damaged and causing paralysis. But I'll also give her an injection of antibiotics to begin the treatment for Lyme disease," said Dr. Riley. "I'll give you some pills that you should give her at home. And

take some of this tick repellent. You just have to use it once a month and it will help keep her free of ticks. The directions are on the box. Don't worry, Elsie will be fine."

"Thanks, doc," said Uncle Fred.

Cats seem to develop Lyme disease less frequently than dogs. This could be because cats groom themselves frequently. A tick may be licked away before it has a chance to bite. But cats can get Lyme disease. So watch for fatigue, listlessness, and joint pain in your cat, too.

Check your pet frequently for ticks. Not only can your dog or cat become infected, it can also bring ticks into the house where they can drop off. They may choose you for their next meal. If you find a tick attached to your pet's skin, remove it with tweezers, just as you would remove it from yourself.

Your dog or cat cannot protect itself. There are now several products available from your veterinarian that will repel ticks. Talk to your vet and find out what he or she recommends. Vaccines are also available for dogs. Again, your vet can give you the most up-to-date information.

Horses

You may not have known that horses can get Lyme disease, too. They can, and it can be a very expensive disease. The cost of veterinarian examinations and tests can be very high. Lyme disease can cause lameness, stiffened and swollen joints, nervous tremors, and hoof inflammation. It can also make your horse extremely sensitive to being touched. This sensitivity may cause a horse to refuse to be saddled.

But not every horse that is infected with Lyme bacteria will actually display symptoms of the disease. This makes diagnosis very difficult.

Blood tests are the first step to diagnosing Lyme disease in horses. But like humans, horses will not test positive until their systems have begun to make antibodies to fight the disease. In many horses, these antibodies are strong enough to keep the disease from causing symptoms. The antibodies are able to fight the disease without the help of medication.

The Lyme Disease Vaccination

Joe lived in New Jersey. He knew that Lyme disease could be very dangerous. When he heard that a Lyme disease vaccination was available, he thought it sounded like a good idea. If the vaccine really prevented Lyme disease, he thought, his whole family should probably get it. Joe had already scheduled an appointment for a physical examination, so he decided to ask his doctor about the vaccine.

Joe waited in an examining room in Dr. Brownstein's office.

"How are you feeling today, Joe?" asked Dr. Brownstein as he walked through the door.

"I feel fine," said Joe. "I just wanted to check things out and be sure everything's really okay."

"The nurse will come in to begin some tests. When she's finished, I'll be back," said Dr. Brownstein.

"Okay," said Joe.

Dr. Brownstein's nurse took blood and a urine sample from Joe. She also gave him an electrocardiogram. She recorded his height and weight. After she left, Joe waited for Dr. Brownstein.

Dr. Brownstein returned and finished the physical. "I'll give you a call if the blood and urine tests show anything unusual," said Dr. Brownstein. "Otherwise, everything looks good. Just lay off those bacon, egg, and cheese sandwiches."

"I have another question," said Joe. "I heard there's a Lyme disease vaccination. My neighbor Pete had Lyme disease and he was sick for a really long time. He had to walk with a cane. I was thinking that I should get the vaccine. Maybe my wife, Kate, and our kids should get it, too. What do you think?"

"The vaccine wasn't tested on young kids, so it's not approved for them," said Dr. Brownstein. "Only adults and teenagers older than fifteen can get it. But I'm not sure it's a great idea anyway. I wouldn't recommend it for either you or Kate."

"Why not?" asked Joe.

"First of all, it's too late in the year. In order for the vaccination to even start to be effective, you have to get two shots, a month apart. The peak season for ticks is right now. By the time you finished with those shots, it would be over. But even then you would only be partly protected. You don't have the full effect of the vaccine until after the third shot. I can't give you that until eleven months after the second shot."

"Three shots! I didn't know I would need three shots," said Joe.

"For the highest level of protection, you need them all," said Dr. Brownstein. "But even then, the vaccine is only 80 percent effective. The studies testing the vaccine were done over only a two-year period. No one knows for sure if the vaccine will keep protecting you longer than that. You may need an annual booster shot."

"When I first heard about the vaccine, I thought it sounded like a good idea," said Joe. "But now I'm not so sure."

"You probably want to wait until more studies are done," said Dr. Brownstein. "You don't really spend a lot of time in the woods. Even with the vaccine, you need to protect yourself against ticks because it's not 100 percent effective. Just be careful and watch for the EM rash. And always tell me about any strange physical symptoms you can't explain."

"Thanks, doc," said Joe. "I guess there's no miracle protection against Lyme disease."

"Not yet," said Dr. Brownstein.

On December 21, 1998, the United States Food and Drug Administration approved a Lyme disease vaccine. This first vaccine, called LYMErix, was not tested on children. As of April 2000, it had not been approved for anyone younger than age fifteen. The vaccine is preventive, protecting against Lyme infection before it occurs.

According to the *New England Journal of Medicine*, the vaccine was tested on nearly 10,000 healthy people ages fifteen to seventy who live in areas where Lyme disease is common. For the highest level of protection, a series of three shots is needed. The first two shots, given a month apart, provide about 50 percent protection. A third shot, given eleven months later, increases protection to about 80 percent (90 percent among people under age sixty-five). Of 5,000 people who received three shots, 13 got Lyme disease compared with 56 of 5,000 people who received "dummy" shots that did not really contain the vaccine.

How the Vaccine Works

According to the American Lyme Disease Foundation, the vaccine protects people from contracting Lyme disease by inducing their bodies to create antibodies that fight the *Borrelia burgdorferi* bacteria. And although there is no solid scientific evidence that you can get Lyme disease from the vaccine, you will test positive for the disease on some of the diagnostic tests. The reason for this is that some of these tests determine whether or not you have the disease by checking for Lyme disease antibodies, which you would then have in your system.

Timing the vaccine is important. You want the protection to be effective during the spring and summer when ticks are most active. Someone who decides to be vaccinated should plan to receive the first two injections in late winter or very early spring, no later than March.

Researchers continue to test the vaccine to make it safe for children. They also hope to develop a vaccine that will work in one dose. The current vaccine, according to Dr. David Volkman, associate professor of medicine and pediatrics at SUNY at Stony Brook, may not be the best choice for most people. First, the highest level of protection is not reached until a year after the first shot. Because the tests were conducted over a two-year period, it is not known if the vaccine works longer than that. It may be necessary to get annual booster shots, similar to an annual flu shot, beginning in the second year to maintain a high level of protection. Also, because the shots are so new, scientists don't know the long-term effects of repeated doses of Lyme vaccine.

Being vaccinated may give you a false sense of security. The vaccine is not 100 percent effective. Even after you have had all three shots, you will still need to take the normal precautions against Lyme disease.

Choosing to Be Vaccinated

Who should consider getting the Lyme disease vaccine? People who live in high-risk areas and spend a lot of time outdoors. If you live in Connecticut, New Jersey, or other Lyme disease "hot spots" and your parents work in jobs that keep them outside, like landscape or utility workers, you may want to talk with them about the vaccine. Also, adults and teenagers over age fifteen in families who enjoy a lot of outdoor activities, like hiking, camping, or hunting, in these areas may choose to be vaccinated. In other places, especially where infected ticks are rarely found, you may want to wait for more research to be conducted. Even those who are vaccinated are not 100 percent protected. You will need to continue to take the same precautions you would if you had not received the vaccine. People considering the vaccine should first talk to their doctors.

Vaccine Side Effects

In December 1999, a lawsuit was filed against SmithKline Beecham, the manufacturers of LYMErix, claiming that doctors were not sufficiently warned about the dangers of the vaccine. The group of people filing the suit allege that the vaccine could trigger a reaction that causes a treatment-resistant Lyme arthritis. This type of arthritis does not respond to antibiotic treatment and cannot be cured. The reaction does not happen to everyone who receives the vaccine. A routine blood test can prove whether an individual is likely to have the reaction before the vaccine is given. The lawsuit claims that SmithKline Beecham did not carefully warn doctors and patients about the possibility of this reaction. Also, the lawsuit claims that SmithKline Beecham did not caution doctors that the vaccine can be dangerous for patients who are already infected with the Lyme bacteria. Investigations are still being conducted to determine whether these claims are valid.

Lyme Disease and Teenagers

Debra sat in the guidance counselor's office at Bethwood High School. She had fallen asleep in Spanish class again. It's no wonder I fall asleep, she thought, Mrs. Allen is so boring. But this had been the second time this week, and Mrs. Allen had sent Debra to the office. The guidance counselor, Miss Welsh, had called Debra's mom.

"While we're waiting for your mom, let's talk a bit, Debra," said Miss Welsh.

"Oh, great," Debra thought.

"This is the second time this week that you've fallen asleep in Mrs. Allen's class," said Miss Welsh. "She also told me that your grades have fallen. And you have forgotten several homework assignments. I've checked with your math and science teachers and they say that you're having similar problems in their classes. Do you have an explanation for this?"

"I don't know," said Debra. "I'm just tired. I fall asleep before I get my homework done."

"Or maybe you're too busy talking with your friends on the phone," said Miss Welsh. "Maybe you spend too much time at the mall."

"No, I don't," said Debra. "Look, you can ask my mom when she gets here. I haven't been to the mall for weeks. And she would know if I was on the phone all the time. I don't mean to fall asleep in class. I don't know why I'm tired all the time."

Debra fought to hold back tears as her mom walked in the door.

"Debra, what's wrong?" asked her mom, Julia. When Debra started crying, Julia looked at Miss Welsh. "Why is Debra here?" Julia asked.

"She fell asleep again during her Spanish class—the second time this week. Her grades have fallen and she doesn't turn in all her homework assignments. Other teachers have the same complaints," said Miss Welsh.

"That's very unusual," said Julia. "Debra has always been a good student. She's very conscientious about her homework."

She put her hand on Debra's shoulder. "Honey, do you feel all right?"

"I'm just so tired all the time," said Debra. "I fall asleep at home, too, when I'm trying to do my home-work. I don't see how I can be so tired when I spend so much time falling asleep."

"I think I'll take Debra home now, Miss Welsh," said Julia. "Please ask her teachers to make a list of the assignments that she has missed. I'll be sure that she gets them done."

"All right," said Miss Welsh.

They left the guidance office and Julia waited while Debra got the books she needed from her locker. As they walked to the car, Julia told Debra that she was going to make an appointment for her at the doctor.

"I don't think it's normal for you to fall asleep at your desk," said Julia. "It's possible that there's some-thing wrong that the doctor can help us with."

"I don't want to go to the doctor. What if she finds something terrible? What if I'm dying?" said Debra.

"I don't think you're dying, honey," Julia said. "But we need to find out what is wrong. Try not to worry."

During adolescence, you will experience physical and psychological changes. Normal teenagers are often rebellious, moody, and irritable. It's the time when you will be looking for your own identity, independent from your parents. As a result, if you complain to your parents or teachers of fatigue, headaches, or stomachaches, your complaints may be attributed to hormonal changes or rebellion. The first reaction of doctors may be to look for emotional or developmental causes for your symptoms.

Debra and Julia waited in Dr. Jessup's examining room. When Dr. Jessup came in, Julia told her about Debra's fatigue problems.

"Fatigue is very common among teenagers," said Dr. Jessup. "Sometimes they say they're tired to avoid being with their parents. They don't want to explain why they're not meeting their responsibilities, so they pretend to fall asleep. Other times, they really are tired, but it's because they stay out late with their friends or because their bodies are growing and changing."

Julia was surprised and insulted by Dr. Jessup's reaction to Debra's symptoms.

"Debra is not purposely avoiding her schoolwork. And she doesn't stay out late with her friends, especially on school nights," said Julia.

"Are you sure?" said Dr. Jessup. "Sometimes kids sneak out without their parents' knowledge."

"Yes, I'm sure," said Julia. "Come on, Debra. We'll find a doctor who is not so quick to dismiss her patient's symptoms."

"I'm just being realistic," said Dr. Jessup. "It is most likely that Debra's fatigue is simply caused by not sleeping at night."

"In this case, that is not the most likely answer," said Julia. "So we need to find someone who is willing to look for medical reasons."

Your parents have probably not recently seen you without your clothes. So, if you find an EM rash, they will not know about it unless you tell them. Many teens hide problems or worries from their parents, hoping the problems will go away by themselves. An EM rash does disappear on its own. The problem appears to be solved. You may believe that your parents will never need to be told.

Randy had a really weird rash under his right arm. It looked red and was a bit bumpy. Every morning, he checked to be sure it was still there. He never told his parents. He figured that they wouldn't know what it was anyway. When he changed for gym, he kept his right arm down as much as possible. He made sure the other kids didn't see his rash.

Finally, one day it seemed to be getting better. Eventually, it went away. I was right, he thought, it was nothing. Good thing I didn't show it to anybody. The other kids would have thought it was really gross.

But then your illness worsens. Untreated Lyme disease creates more, seemingly mysterious, symptoms. Without knowledge of the rash, your parents and doctor will not be able to accurately attribute your physical and emotional symptoms to Lyme disease. They will not understand why you are tired all the time. They will have no defense against teachers who blame your falling grades on laziness or defiance.

You may feel helpless, too. You also notice the changes and don't know why they are happening.

Be Honest About Your Symptoms

Jessica was sick, but she didn't know it. She was tired all the time. She hated being around people, especially her parents. She always seemed to have a headache.

Jessica came home from school and went straight to her room, shutting the door. Her mom, Anne, knocked on the door.

"Jessica, are you all right?" Anne asked.

"I'm fine. I'm just tired," Jessica said. She was lying on the bed and did not get up to open the door.

"Can I come in?" asked Anne.

"What for? I said, I'm fine," Jessica answered.

"Are you sure nothing's wrong? Do you feel okay?" Anne tried again.

"Nothing's wrong. I feel fine," said Jessica. But she was not fine. She had another severe headache. She couldn't stand to have the lights on. She didn't want her mom to know that she was lying in the dark, so she didn't let her in.

Jessica was scared. She didn't know why she felt this way. But she was more afraid that she would find out that she had a deadly disease, like cancer. If she never told her parents how she felt, they would not make her go to the doctor.

If you have been bitten by a tick or you have had an EM rash, tell your parents immediately. First, they will be relieved. Knowledge of the rash will make the diagnosis much easier. Treatment can begin sooner.

But if you have kept your secret for a long time, it may be a while before the treatment brings results. The symptoms may return and require additional medication. Hopefully, you will find that much of your stress is relieved simply by finding the cause of your problems. You are not crazy. You are not dying. Your Lyme disease can be treated. But only if you are honest with your parents and your doctor.

In areas of the country where Lyme disease occurs often, doctors will probably know how to recognize and treat the symptoms. School officials will also be more sympathetic once they are told of your diagnosis. However, in areas where Lyme disease is more rare, you and your parents may have more difficulty getting an accurate diagnosis. Teachers and school administrators may not understand how long recovery can take. You and your parents must work together to get the help you need.

Lyme Disease and Substance Abuse

Ron and Alice Morgan were worried about their daughter Jayne. Jayne had always been a cheerful, outgoing girl. In her sophomore year, she was elected vice president of her class. She was the sports editor of the school newspaper.

But Jayne had changed. She was moody and irritable. She snapped at everyone for no apparent reason. She spent most of her time at home alone in her room. Sometimes she refused to eat.

At school, her grades had fallen. Jayne never seemed to do any homework. She no longer worked on the school paper. Jayne said that she had quit because it was "stupid." Alice, however, suspected that Jayne had been asked to give up her job because she was not making deadlines.

Ron and Alice had arranged a meeting with Jayne's guidance counselor, Mr. Oswald. They had not told Jayne about it. They hated going behind her back. But they were afraid of her reaction.

"I don't know what to do," said Alice to Mr. Oswald. "When I ask Jayne if something is bothering her, she yells 'leave me alone' and storms into her room, slamming the door. We're both very worried about her, but we can't find out anything from her. Do you have a suggestion?"

"We've noticed the change in Jayne, too," said Mr. Oswald. "Her teachers are finding her uncooperative and withdrawn. That's a big change from last year. By any chance, have you taken Jayne to the doctor?"

"No," said Alice. "Not recently. She has always been very healthy."

"It's possible that there are physical reasons for Jayne's behavior," said Mr. Oswald. "If she had symptoms she can't explain, she may be trying to hide them from you by pushing you away. She could be scared, too. The stress caused by her anxiety could

be keeping her awake at night. She may be tired during the day, making her more irritable."

"It would actually be a relief to find a physical explanation for the changes in Jayne," said Ron.

"There is another possibility," said Mr. Oswald.

"What's that?" asked Alice.

"We should consider the possibility that Jayne is using drugs," said Mr. Oswald.

"Jayne would never do that," said Ron.

"I hope you're right," said Mr. Oswald. "But I would suggest that you have the doctor do a drug test, just to be on the safe side. We're not trying to accuse Jayne of anything. We want to help her."

"We'll make an appointment with the doctor right away," said Alice.

One of the biggest concerns in the United States and Canada is teen alcohol and drug abuse. Many schools provide expert speakers to help parents deal with this problem. News reports tell of teens who are killed while driving drunk. Television advertising warns parents to be alert for the telltale signs of substance abuse.

Unfortunately, many of these signs—social withdrawal, suddenly failing grades, fatigue, confusion, memory loss—are also symptoms of Lyme disease. In fear, your parents may ask you to take a drug screening test. You may feel insulted or even threatened by this request. But remember, your parents are not trying to prove that you are taking drugs. They want to show that you are not taking drugs. Then you, your parents, and your doctor can work together to treat the real cause of your problems.

Academic Performance

Alex was planning a career in medicine. He hoped to go to Harvard. In high school, he had always made the honor roll. At least until this year. During the summer, a tick infected with Lyme disease had bitten Alex. His illness had not been discovered right away. He had not received treatment until his forgetfulness and lack of concentration had made his grades fall. He had also missed a lot of school.

This could not have happened at a worse time, Alex thought. How am I ever going to get into Harvard now?

The arthritis or flulike symptoms of Lyme disease may force you to stay home and miss valuable school time. Headaches and fatigue can reduce your attention span and make it difficult to concentrate on homework. You may find it difficult to focus. On top of already high stress levels, you may feel out of control. You may feel that your chances of being accepted to college are slipping away as your grades fall.

Lyme disease can be especially devastating if it attacks during your junior year in high school. Your grades are especially important during this year. You are preparing college applications and taking SAT and advanced placement tests.

Although your grades may suffer because of your illness, you do not need to give up your college plans. Once you understand that Lyme disease is the cause of your symptoms, you can regain control over your life. Ask your doctor to write a letter of recommendation, explaining the unusual circumstances that affected your grades. The letter should also show that your health has improved and is no longer affecting your scholastic performance.

Lyme Disease and Learning Disabilities

While Lyme disease is not actually a learning disability, the physical symptoms, especially those caused by Stage III Lyme disease, can make learning more difficult. In extreme cases, these difficulties may be classified as learning disabilities. Under the Americans with Disabilities Act (ADA) and the Rehabilitation Act of 1973, students with learning disabilities are guaranteed equal access to programs and services. You may be eligible for special accommodations. However, a qualified professional must document the learning disability. Qualified professionals include educational psychologists, school psychologists, neurophysiologists, learning disability specialists, and medical doctors with special training in the effects of illness on learning. The professional will use tests to evaluate the impact that your disability has on your academic ability. He or she will make a specific diagnosis and recommendations for special services that may be necessary to help you learn. According to the Association on Higher Education and Disability (AHEAD), a clinical summary that includes the following information should be provided to your school:

⇨ The evaluator should demonstrate that other causes for your academic problems, such as lack of motivation, emotional problems, language difficulties, or poor educational background have been ruled out.

➥ The evaluator should show how patterns in your learning progress reflect the presence of a learning disability. For example, falling grades that can be traced to the onset of Lyme disease symptoms could demonstrate a pattern.

➥ The evaluator should show a substantial limitation to learning caused by the disability.

➥ The evaluator should show why specific accommodations are needed and how they will affect your specific disability. Such accommodations could include extended time taking tests.

Your school has a responsibility to respect your privacy and keep these reports confidential. No information about you may be released without your written consent.

Lyme Disease and the Scholastic Aptitude Test (SAT)

What about the SATs? How can you do your best on the SAT if you are suffering with Lyme disease?

The Educational Testing Service, the organization that oversees the administration of the Scholastic Aptitude Test, has recognized that students with chronic Lyme disease may be eligible for a special, extended-time test. You must provide documentation from a qualified professional to show that you need this accommodation. You may be required to take an evaluation test to show how your Lyme disease has limited your academic ability. You may also need to provide the history of your illness, including school reports and medical history. Complete information about requirements for special testing accommodations are available from the corporate headquarters of the Educational Testing Service, Rosedale Road, Princeton, NJ, 08541, (609) 921-9000. You can also use the ETS Web site: *http://www.ets.org.*

The Last Word on Lyme Disease

Claire Lipton's parents drove her home from the hospital. They had rented a wheelchair for Claire to use until her knees recovered. Ed stopped the car in the driveway, brought the wheelchair up to the car, and helped Claire climb into it.

"I feel like such a baby," said Claire.

"Don't be silly, honey," said Suzanne. "Being sick does not make you a baby. Your Lyme disease is not your fault."

"Okay, but how long will I have to stay in this wheelchair?" Claire asked.

"The doctor said it could be anywhere from a couple of days to three weeks," said Ed. "Basically, it depends on how long your knees keep hurting. You'll know when you don't need the wheelchair. When you can walk, you won't have to ride."

As Ed pushed Claire toward the front door, their neighbor Dan rode by on his bike. "Hi, Claire," he called and waved. Then he turned his bike and rode up the Lipton's driveway.

"What's up with the wheelchair?" asked Dan. "Why can't you walk?"

"I have Lyme disease," said Claire. "It made my knees swell up. They hurt so much that I can't walk."

"Wow," said Dan. "How long will you have to stay in that thing?"

"I'm not sure," said Claire. "They gave me antibiotics in the hospital. My knees already hurt less. I think I will be able to get up pretty soon."

"I hope so," said Dan. "It must be pretty boring just sitting in that chair."

"No kidding," said Claire. "Dad, can I stay outside? I won't feel so cooped up."

"Sure, honey," said Ed.

Claire was lucky. In a few days, her knees were much better. Soon she and Dan were taking turns racing down the driveway in her wheelchair. Fortunately, she, her parents, and her doctor had recognized her Lyme disease in time to treat it.

Lyme disease can be very dangerous. You can lessen the danger by protecting yourself when you are outside in a place where ticks live. Wear long sleeves, long pants, socks, and closed shoes when hiking or playing in the woods or in tall grass. Clear litter, brush, and long grass from around your home. Consider removing woodpiles and stone walls.

Check yourself for ticks when you come inside. If you see a red, spreading EM rash on your skin, tell your parents and go to the doctor right away. Start treatment as soon as you can.

You may be infected with Lyme disease even though you have never had the EM rash. Swollen joints, especially knees, headaches, and achiness are symptoms of disseminated Lyme disease. Disseminated Lyme disease can lead to more serious symptoms. If you live in an area where deer ticks are found, it is smart to understand all the symptoms of Lyme disease.

Remember, if Lyme disease is diagnosed early, it is almost always easily treated and cured. Hiding your symptoms will only make the problem worse. Talk to your parents or guidance counselor if you think you may have Lyme disease. If you find a tick attached to your body or see an EM rash, tell your parents or make an appointment to see your doctor right away. Early detection and prevention are the best ways to avoid the more debilitating symptoms of this disease that continues to baffle the medical community.

Glossary

antibiotic A medicine used to treat Lyme disease and other diseases caused by bacteria.

antibodies The cells in your body that fight off bacteria that cause disease.

arthritis Swollen and painful joints. This is a symptom of Stage II, or disseminated, Lyme disease.

Bell's palsy A symptom of Stage II, or disseminated, Lyme disease. Muscles on one side of the face become paralyzed and cause that side of the face to look droopy.

Borrelia burgdorferi The bacteria that causes Lyme disease.

chronic Lyme disease (Stage III Lyme disease) This is the most dangerous form of Lyme disease and can include heart and liver problems. Chronic Lyme disease is more common in adults and is relatively rare in children.

disseminated Lyme disease The second stage of Lyme disease, when the bacteria has spread throughout the body and causes symptoms like arthritis and Bell's palsy.

erythema migrans Often called the EM rash, it is the most common symptom of early Lyme disease. The rash is lighter in the center, around the bite wound. Red rings expand outward giving this rash its nickname, the "bull's eye" rash.

host The animal or human off of which a tick feeds.

larva The second stage of a tick's life cycle, the time when it has six legs and is very tiny.

molt To shed an old body structure in order to form a new one. A tick changes body form, or molts, during three of its four stages of life.

multiple sclerosis A disease that attacks the nervous system and is sometimes confused with Stage III Lyme disease.

nymph The third stage of a tick's life cycle. At this time it is the size of a poppy seed and has eight legs. You are most likely to become infected with Lyme disease from a tick in the nymph stage of life.

parasites Animals or insects that live off of other animals, or hosts. They depend on the hosts for survival.

spirochete A spiral-shaped bacteria, like the *Borrelia burgdorferi* bacteria, which causes Lyme disease.

symptom A sign that you may have a disease. An EM rash is a symptom of Lyme disease.

Where to Go for Help

In the United States

American Lyme Disease Foundation
Mill Pond Offices
293 Route 100
Somers, NY 10589
(914) 277-6970
Web site: http://aldf.com

Lyme Alliance
P.O. Box 454
Concord, MI 49237
(517) 563-3582
Web site: http://www.lymealliance.org

Lyme Disease Foundation, Inc.
One Financial Plaza, 18th Floor
Hartford, CT 06103
(800) 886-LYME (5963)
Web site: http://www.lyme.org

Lyme Disease Network
43 Winton Road
East Brunswick, NJ 08816
Web site: http://www.lymenet.org

National Institutes of Health
NIAID Office of Communications and Public Liaison
Building 31, Room 7A-50
31 Center Drive MSC 2520
Bethesda, MD 20892-2520
Web site: http://www.niaid.nih.gov/publications/tick.htm

In Canada

Canadian Infectious Disease Society
2197 Promenade Riverside Drive, Suite 504
Pebb Building
Ottawa, ON K1H 7X3
(613) 260-3233
Web site: http://www.cids.medical.org

Health Canada
Laboratory Centre for Disease Control
Bureau of Infectious Diseases
Tunney's Pasture
AL 0913A
Ottawa, ON K1A 0K9
(613) 957-2991
Web site: http://www.hc-sc.gc.ca

Tick Testing Centers

BBI North American Clinical Laboratories
75 North Mountain Road
New Britain, CT 06053
(800) 866-NALG (6254)

IGeneX, Inc.
797 San Antonio Road
Palo Alto, CA 94303
(800) 832-3200
Web site: http://www.igenex.com

Iowa State University
Department of Entomology
Lyme Disease Project
440 Science II
Ames, IA 50011-3222
Web site: http://www.ent.iastate.edu/lds/lds.html

Lyme Alert Tick Test
1110 Somerset Street
New Brunswick, NJ 08901
(732) 249-0148

University of Rhode Island
Fisheries, Animal, and Veterinary Science Department
Tick Research Laboratory
127 Woodward Hall
Kingston, RI 02881-0816
(401) 874-2547
Web site: http://www.riaes.org/resources/ticklab

For Further Reading

Barbour, Alan G. *Lyme Disease: The Cause, the Cure, the Controversy.* Baltimore: Johns Hopkins University Press, 1996.

Donnelly, Karen. *Everything You Need to Know About Lyme Disease.* New York: Rosen Publishing Group, 2000.

Lang, Denise V., and Joseph Territo. *Coping with Lyme Disease: A Practical Guide to Dealing with Diagnosis and Treatment.* (2nd ed.) New York: Henry Holt and Co., 1997.

Murray, Polly. *The Widening Circle: A Lyme Disease Pioneer Tells Her Story.* New York: Saint Martin's Press, 1996.

Rahn, Daniel W., and Janine Evans. *Lyme Disease.* Philadelphia: American College of Physicians, 1998.

Vanderhoof-Forschner, Karen. *Everything You Need to Know About Lyme Disease and Other Tick-Borne Disorders.* New York: John Wiley & Sons, 1997.

Index

F

family (parents, siblings),
27, 31, 34, 78
fatigue, 1, 17, 24, 31, 38,
82, 87, 88
fever, 1, 11, 24, 37

H

headaches, 1, 3, 11, 14,
17, 38, 82, 88, 93
hearing, problems with, 17
heart, 22–25
heartbeat, irregular or
erratic, 18, 23

I

immune system, 22, 48
infection, 1, 2, 3, 7, 14,
24, 40, 41, 56,
76, 93
insecticides, 63–64
insect repellent, 60

J

joint pain/swollen joints,
1, 3, 5, 6, 13,
38, 93

K

knee pain, 5, 13, 21, 93

L

learning disabilities, 89
Lyme anxiety, 34–37
Lyme carditis, 22–25
Lyme, Connecticut, 5, 6
Lyme disease
academic
performance, effect
on, 27, 88–89
in animals, 69–73
and children, 12–13,
60, 77
diagnosis of, 5, 8, 12,
13, 17, 38–45, 48,
56, 85, 94
discovery of, 6–7, 21
how you get it, 7, 9,
39–40, 57
and pregnancy, 2, 60
psychological aspects
of, 26–37
Stage 1, 9–12, 40, 47
Stage 2/disseminated,
12–18, 38, 47, 48
Stage 3/chronic,
20–22, 27, 32, 38,
42, 47, 48, 89
symptoms of, 1, 3,
10–25, 38, 85, 87, 93
and teenagers, 80–91
testing for, 5, 24,
40–43
treatment of, 7, 22,
25, 39, 46–51, 85

V

vaccination, 76–79
vision problems, 5, 17
vomiting, 17

W

walking, problems with,
    5, 13, 21